"You're So Lucky"

"You're So Lucky"

Grace Ash Wethor

ISBN-10: 1985034433
ISBN-13: 978-1985034433

In memory of Amber.
This amazing young woman had an enthusiasm for life, a passion for people, and a smile to light up the room.

CONTENTS

8

ACKNOWLEDGMENTS

From the bottom of my heart, I want to thank the survivors, fighters, families, and angels who were brave enough to share their stories and words of wisdom. Thank you to the illustrators who dove inside my mind and made my vision come to life. Last but not least, thank you to everyone who has supported me these past three years. You are truly the reason I was able to write this book and call myself a survivor.

10

Lucky

A lot of people tell me "you're so lucky" after they hear my story. Well okay, first they say "OMG, I'm so sorry" and then they say "you're so lucky." But what is luck anyways? Would you have told me I was lucky three years ago when I was literally given a death sentence? Luck is defined as success or failure apparently brought by chance rather than through one's own actions. In other words random. But I don't think this was random...how could it be? That was when I decided to be in control of my "luck." You are probably thinking "Grace, that's not how it works." But, why not? It's your life. Make it that way.

<u>DAY 1 OF 1095</u>

You never think it will happen to you.

"No way I'll fail this test."

"No way I'll get the flu."

"No way I'll get cancer…."

This was the "invincible superhero" mindset that I lived with my entire childhood. I never thought something like this would happen to me. I knew I was different, but I never knew how.

That was until one day in 7th grade. I had been tired and sick for a while, but no one could figure out why. A lot of people told me I was depressed, just a teenager, or making it up for attention.

One day they did a blood test and realized my red and white blood cell count was off (a marker for Leukemia) and they sent me to the Children's Hospital Of Minneapolis. I was checked into the Hematology Department. There they took even more blood and did hundreds of test. The doctors very quickly realized that I didn't have Leukemia. The next six months of my life were spent trying to figure out why I had symptoms for Leukemia, but I didn't actually have Leukemia.

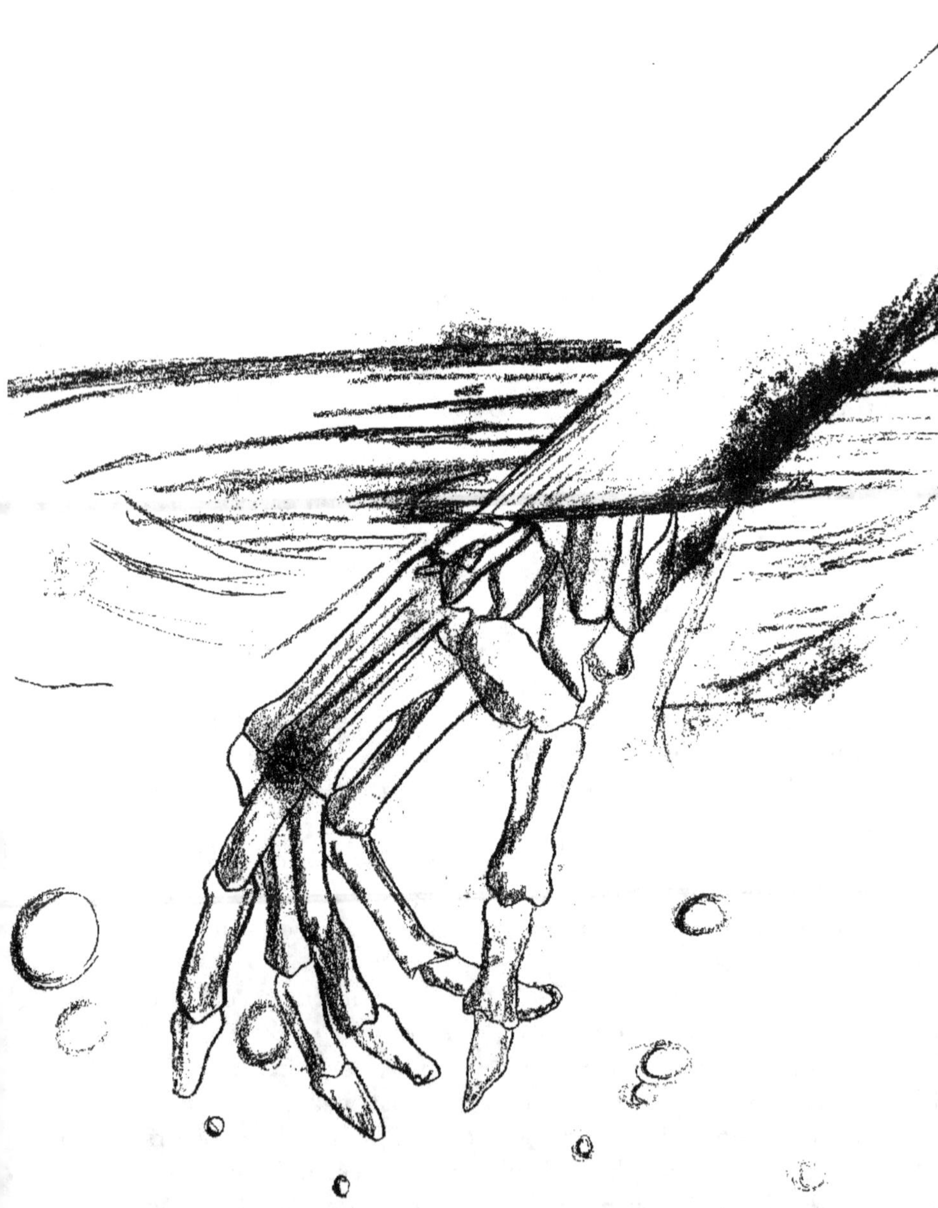

In Between
By Grace Wethor

January 9th, 2015

I wake up dreading going to the doctor's office again. I had been at the same dismal hospital for the past week and was getting tired of the bland food.

I get dressed and we start the drive through snowy Uptown Minneapolis in freezing -7 degree weather.

We park in our usual spot and head into the hospital. Winding through the familiar barren hallways all the way to the imaging department.

I had never had an MRI before.

A lady takes my arm and places yet another hospital band on my wrist and we head back to a room. A male nurse comes in and tells me some bad joke that I can't even remember (he tells it every time). He draws my blood and gives me an IV port.

I'm handed a beat-up black binder full of movie choices. I pick Elf.

Jump to 3 hours later.
Yes.
Three hours…
In a 2 foot by 2 foot tube…
With the loudest beeping noise you have ever heard…

I change back into my gym clothes and we head out the large revolving door. I was on my way back to school and it was time for P.E. class. We were doing the dance unit, which of course, was my favorite.

But I didn't make it to gym class that day.

We drove down the highway.

Down the street.

Down the driveway.

And up to the front door of the school.

Through the glass window I could see the receptionist.

My mom's phone rings.

It's a quick call.

5

10

seconds.

I get ready to get out of the car, but the car doesn't stop. We keep driving.

Down the driveway.

Down the street.

Down the highway.

And back up to the front door of the hospital.

Once inside, my mom was taken one way and I was taken to a cabana, basically a three walled room. There a nurse took my blood pressure, weighed me, and measured how tall I was.

Even though she had done it just a couple hours earlier.

She then asked me a question that I still have a hard time answering to this day.

"On a scale of **1** to **10**, how much pain are you in right now?"

1 - 2 - 3 - 4 - 5 - 6 - 7 - 8 - 9 - 10

Now think about it…

You're not bleeding and your limbs are all attached so you're fine. Right?

For the past six months of my life, people had been telling me I was making up my pain. Was I? Was I really just a 1 and it was all in my head?
Unfortunately it was the opposite situation. I had been feeling the pain for so long that I had started to numb it.

I look up.

A **5** I guess…

You know how you hear your own name so much that sometimes you imagine someone saying it. Well that's what that day felt like that. Except it wasn't my imagination.

MY NAME WAS EVERYWHERE.

WETHOR, GRACE A

FEMALE, AGE: 13

All of a sudden every nurse, every doctor, every person in this hospital was walking past my room quietly whispering my name. To colleagues, on paperwork, into walkie talkies. Everywhere.

Finally, after what seemed like hours of waiting, a nurse took me to another room.

Inside I would find my missing mother.

She was smiling.

But it was the smile someone gave when you could tell that they had been crying.

Not long after that, a doctor came in, a new one, and she showed me a picture of my brain.

That day I was diagnosed with a Brain Stem Glioma, a type of tumor in the Brain Stem. Because of the location, surgery was not an option and chemotherapy/radiation has a slim chance of working. So I went home.

8% chance of survival over the upcoming 6 months with no treatment.

37% chance of survival over one year with treatment.
(Keep in mind no traditional treatment is even available for my type of tumor…)

20% chance of survival over two years.

13% chance of survival over three years.

Would I be a part of that *lucky* 13%?

I guess you could say this is where my LUCK started.

I don't really remember the rest of the day.

It was like I was in a *dream*…

Or a nightmare,

I wasn't sure yet.

However, I knew one thing. I didn't have control over this thing that had happened to me but it was time to make a decision and head out on my next big adventure.

Growing up I was a super active kid. I was a world champion synchronized figure skater. I was a trapeze performer in the circus. I was on a dance team. The list just goes on and on. I was always looking for the next crazy thing I could accomplish. At that moment in my life, I knew it was time for Los Angeles.

I had been passionate about modeling and acting for a longtime, but I decided it was finally time to pursue it as a full-time career.

This book is basically an unedited diary full of poems, stories, sketches and excerpts from my time in L.A. This is my path to becoming a part of the lucky 13% of three-year Brain Stem Glioma survivors.

So, um, good news…
The fact that you are reading this right now means I survived the original six month time period. YAAAAY. That's cool lol.

I recently celebrated the three-year anniversary of my diagnosis and officially became a part of the Lucky 13% club. So double YAAAAY.

I finally felt like it was time to share an inside look to the time where I wasn't so sure if I would be in this "club" or not.

So here we go.

Welcome to "You're So Lucky."

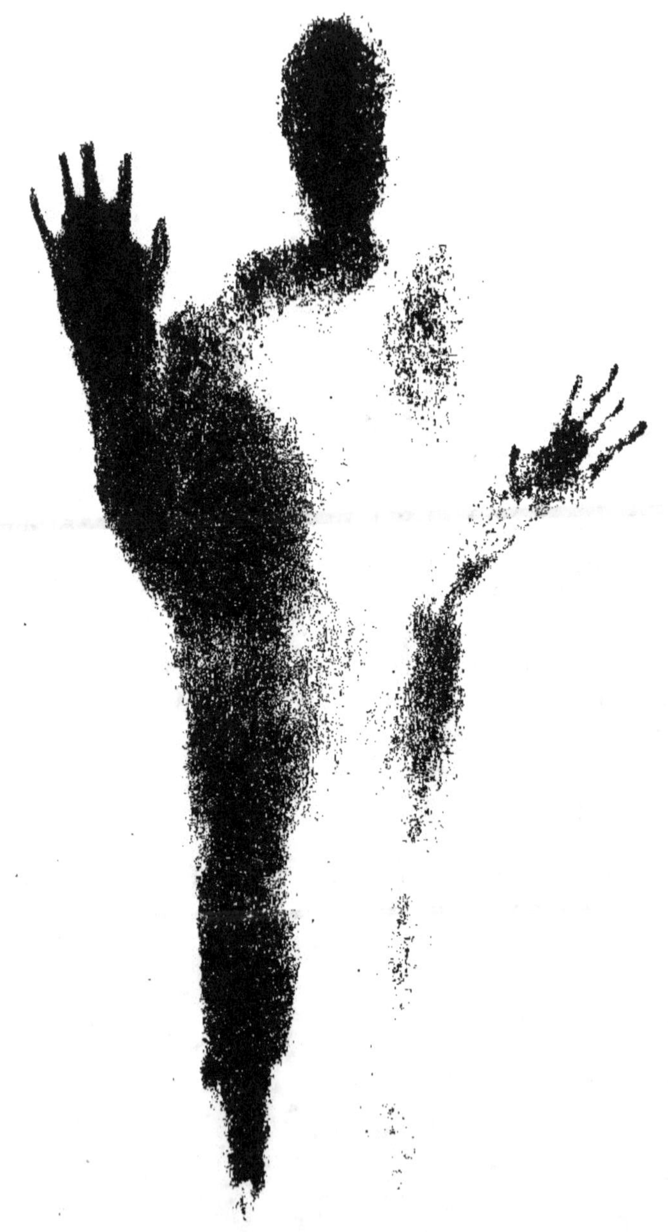

Through The Glass
By Grace Wethor

white wall

i stare at it
it doesn't move
i stare some more
the white wall huddled in the left
corner of the storage room

at first glance the wall is white
tall
blank

you can tell the wall has been hidden
behind mountains of memories for a long
time...
too long

i step closer
the obscure wall sits

upon closer inspection i can tell

i see the scratches and the marks
the dents and bumps
on the no longer blank
white wall

shirley temples

do you remember those days
when we sat at the beach
in those uncomfortable lawn chairs

we drank Shirley Temples
with mountains of cherries
and our biggest worry was the
8% chance of rain

but then the cherries shriveled
and the sprite went flat
the waves settled
and the tide swept our minds away

oh how I long to sit in those
uncomfortable lawn chairs
once again

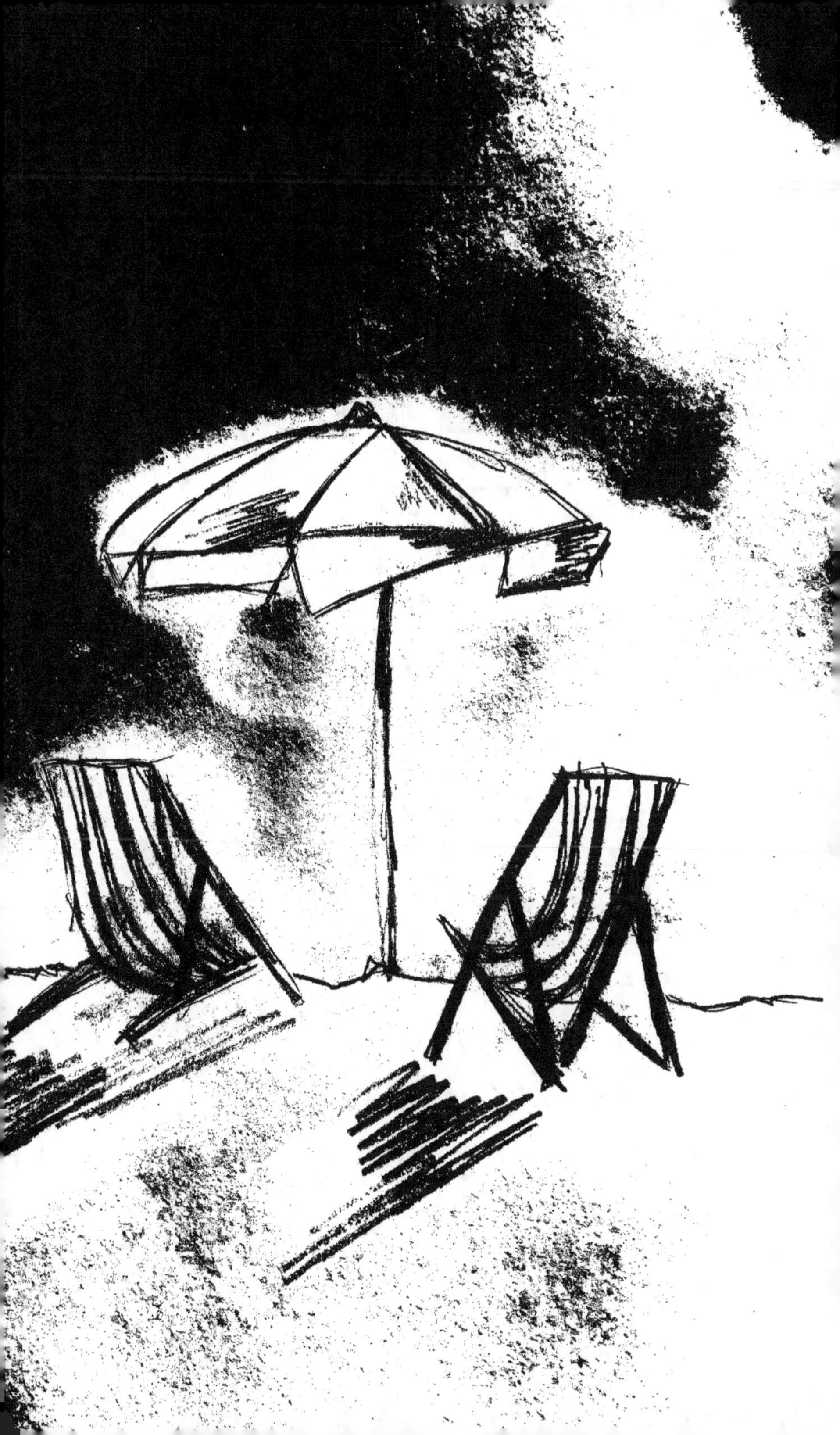

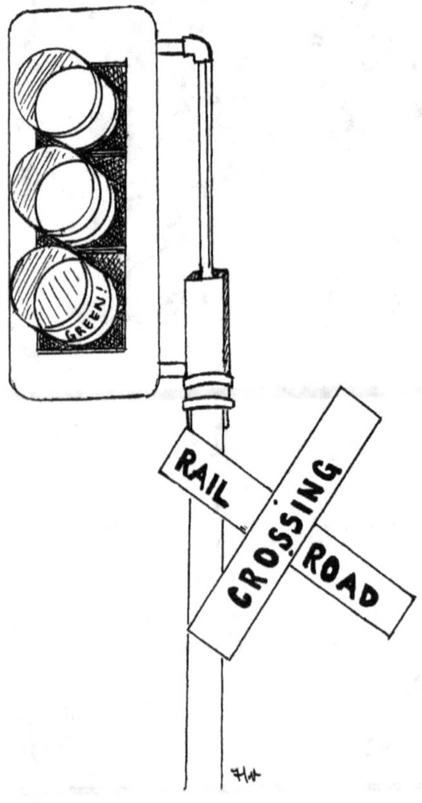

Sketch By Heather Rosati

Yellow Lights

but we are young
we are dumb
we're lighting matches on our tongues

we're talking about the past
breaking glass
the yellow lights tell us drive fast

When writing this book, I realized that there was something missing. Then it hit me, it was a sense of community. Throughout my journey, the brain tumor community contributed so much to my learning and growing as a survivor and fighter. That was why I decided to have Author Chapter Takeovers.

Throughout this book, different people in the community affected by brain tumors in different ways will contribute their thoughts as well as stories.

enjoy.

Gabrielle Camacho

Pineal Cystic Tumor Survivor

Gabrielle

Tina the Tumor

In 2013 I was diagnosed with a Pineal Cyst. Later, I was to find out it was a benign tumor. I was taking track at the time and one day I started to get a headache and weird vision problems. I looked up at my coach and could only see half of him, as if part of him was cut out of a magazine. I could see the background, but half of him was pitch black. My mom was worried about my vision and took me to a neurologist. This doctor ended up being the first of many. He had me walk around a room and do some tests and then we talked about my symptoms. He ordered an MRI, which is basically a big white machine with a hole in the middle that is really loud. Finally, about a month later, we returned and he informed up that I had a Pineal Cyst. He explained that the cyst probably had nothing to do with what was happening to me, and that these kinds of cysts can cause problems, but only if they are much larger. To monitor it I had to do MRIs every year. I was very reluctant towards having the MRIs, I had to have contrast where they stuck a needle in my veins. I found it very painful and it felt as if heat was coursing through my veins. For the next few years I had headaches frequently, yet nothing else to cause concern.

Two years later, it was the beginning of eighth grade and I was in my dance class. We were working on a new dance for our showcase and I started to have my "episodes". These episodes consisted of me losing control of my upper body, my head would fall forward, my jaw would drop, my hands would curl up, I couldn't speak, but I was conscious. They lasted for anywhere from a couple of seconds up to a minute, and though they were pretty easy to hide, I was growing very self-conscious. At first I thought it was a one-time thing, but it kept persisting in that class when we started to dance. I told my close friend who was in the class with me and we discussed it at lunch with our other two friends. They didn't understand and I felt like an alien. I finally got up the courage to tell my mom and once I did she started to notice them. They would happen when I would get out of the car and then started to happen all the time, when I was laying down, standing up, and when I would begin to walk or run. The episodes became progressively worse, and I started to have more symptoms like fatigue, headaches, reflux, and more. We went back to see my neurologist and it was like listening to a recording. "Your symptoms can't be related to the cyst. The cyst is too small to cause any problems." I was furious, doctors are supposed to help you try and figure out what is wrong with you and help find solutions. Instead he was telling me it was all in my head. I felt belittled and demeaned.

My mother was not happy with what the doctor had to say, so she made an appointment for me to see another doctor in Los Angeles, only it would take me 6 months to get in. So as I waited things got worse and I started having these episodes multiple times a day. I feared my peers would see right through me, think I was a freak, or worse, making it up. Finally, we met with my new neurologist, Dr. Tavyev. She researched my symptoms extensively and found a case study that sounded similar to my episodes. Dr. Tavyev thought I may have narcolepsy with cataplexy and gave us information on it, and also scheduled for me to have a sleep study to see if this was the problem. I was over the moon with excitement, I was going to find out what was wrong with me! It had to be narcolepsy with cataplexy, I finally had an answer. A couple weeks later I had the sleep study done. My mother and I arrived at the building around sunset. When I got to my room I changed into a hospital gown and then a technician proceeded to hook me up to a bunch of cords with glue. I slept for a couple of hours and then they would wake me up for a couple of hours and the process would repeat itself. A few weeks later the doctor explained that the test came out negative, but if I had trouble sleeping I could come back for more tests. My spirits came crashing down so fast. I was angry. I no longer had an answer, I was back to square one. I was so close, but my journey was far from over.

At that point, my mom and I were convinced that my symptoms were caused by this Pineal Cystic tumor. During her research my mom came across a support group for parents who have kids with Pineal Cysts. A specific doctor kept coming up and he was based in Texas. He was one of the few doctors that had performed many surgeries on people with this type of cystic tumor. I was skeptical at first, so one of the support group ladies put me in contact with a survivor that had undergone surgery. This girl was amazing. She answered all my questions and put my mind at ease. We discussed her symptoms and found out we had a lot of them in common. She explained her experience of recovery from the surgery. After talking to her I made the decision to tell my mom I would like to try the surgery. My mom quickly sent my records, MRIs and information over to the neurosurgeon in Texas. He is one of the few neurosurgeons that will work on my particular tumor. We then anxiously waited for a consultation date.

My parents and I headed to Houston, Texas for my consultation and met with Dr. Kim on November 8, 2016. We stayed with my uncle and aunt who live only an hour away from the doctor's office. Finally, we went to the doctor's office about an hour before my consultation to meet other girls with the same diagnosis and their families that my mom had connected with online. The online group calls the girls with Pineal Cysts Cysters. I was nervous to meet them all, but they were so kind as we shared stories and experiences about other doctors. I was extremely quiet, but listened intently. The first girl I met, Megan, had already had surgery and was getting her stitches out. The second girl I met, Makemma, was there for her consultation as well. Another, Aynalem, also had surgery and was going home.

One thing I can tell you is that these girls are warriors. They were fearless going through something so scary, brain surgery. After our get-together, we all had our appointments. We were the last ones called back, and my parents and I anxiously followed the nurse into a room where we waited. Eventually a consultant came in and asked us various questions. He made it sound like I wasn't going to be eligible for surgery and I was terrified. He left the room and came back with the doctor a few minutes later. The doctor introduced himself and we restated what we had told the consultant. Then the most miraculous thing happened. He said he thought I would benefit from the surgery. My heart skipped a beat. Was I really going to get better? Did I really have a chance at being normal? I was euphoric. I was officially set to have surgery on December 7, 2016.

Now I had almost a month before surgery and I had to watch a video to prepare. In the video, something the doctor said stuck with me: he said that my Pineal Cyst was a tumor. That may not seem like a big thing, but it is. When he referred to it as a tumor it made it more real to me. I now had an answer, and not only an answer but a way to fix the problem. Before going back to Houston for surgery we told my family and friends what was going on in more depth. There were mixed reactions. Some didn't understand, some were scared, some didn't think surgery was the way to go, but everyone supported me. My mom and I decided to name my tumor and came up with "Tina", after a character from one of our favorite movies, Napoleon Dynamite. The day before my mom and I were going to leave, my family came over to say their goodbyes and wish me good luck. I spent my "goodbyes" reassuring them that I would be okay. I understood that they were nervous, but I was excited to no longer be in pain.

The next day we departed for Houston. Upon arrival my uncle and aunt picked us up to take us to our rented apartment near the medical center. I had pre OP appointments Monday and Tuesday explaining what my surgery would entail and how I should prepare. I was nervous, but never afraid. My dad had flown in on Tuesday. On Wednesday, the morning of my surgery, we waited with anticipation. We were all very tired and waited a while for the nurse to take me to a room. When she did we waited some more, then another nurse took me to the operating room. The ride to the operation room was bumpy and the fluorescent lights hurt my eyes. The anesthesiologist put me to sleep and surgery began. I remember waking up when it was over, I was in a room with other patients and I heard noises. My eyes were closed for some reason and I couldn't open them. My parents came in to see me shortly after and I grabbed my dad's hand. I felt safe.

Though it was far from easy, recovery could begin. I spent two nights in the hospital, and then they sent me to the apartment near the medical center. I needed help walking and going to the restroom, I couldn't speak in full sentences for about five days, and I was in immense pain with headaches. I would take naps throughout the day, but every time I woke up my head felt like it was going to explode. The doctor said walking would help with my headaches, yet I didn't believe it; I could barely stand up on my own let alone walk. Yet through my doubts my parents insisted it was possible. They would patiently hold my hand and brace my back as I walked extremely slow. We walked back and forth in the parking lot over and over. By the second week I could walk on my own, so I attempted to make a sandwich one afternoon. I was so emotional because it took all of my energy to make that sandwich. To toast the bread, spread the mayo, add cheese and chicken, was exhausting. Making sandwiches is virtually the easiest thing in the world, but for some reason I had a difficult time with it. That simple moment was when I realized I was going to have to learn how to do some things all over again. A few weeks later I had my stitches removed, which hurt so much, but the following day we went home and said goodbye to Houston.

The day we returned home my dad took me out to lunch to see some of my family. I will never forget my

Grandpa's face. He lit up when he saw me and I was so happy to see him! On Christmas I got to see the rest of my family and they were all so caring and understanding. I didn't have a lot of energy so I had to rest a lot. I also had really bad headaches for a couple of months and my fatigue was still there. At first it was frustrating how long it was taking, but I accepted it over time. I was gradually getting better and about eighty percent of my symptoms were gone. If I had headaches they were easily subdued by ibuprofen, yet I still had the episodes and fatigue.

I didn't start school again until three months post-op. It was a bit stressful, but I passed all my classes. That year I didn't see much of my friends because I was homeschooled, and when I wasn't doing school I was resting and had little energy. I felt isolated from the world and for a while I was okay with it! Then I found myself feeling lonely. I had no one to talk to or hangout with. Then one day I had to go to school for mandatory science labs and I met Grace who also has a brain tumor. I was shocked and asked her what kind and then told her I had had a brain tumor too. We instantly bonded over our shared experiences with doctors and how we explained it to other people. She invited me to go with her to a camp for children with brain tumors in Montana, and we ended up staying in the same cabin.

We attended camp in the summer of 2017. It was terrifying, because I had never been to another state without at least one of my parents, but I was also excited for this experience. I also invited Megan, one of the cysters I had met at my consultation. I arrived in Montana and the bus ride to the campsite was beautiful. There were trees everywhere and it was so green, it was all so new and exciting. I was uncomfortable at first, but once I started to trust the others I made some friends. We bonded over similar experiences and how we weren't always treated fairly by others. We laughed and we cried. We sang camp songs and we conquered fears. There was hiking, horseback riding, games, art, zip lining, archery, rafting and so much more. I can tell you all these beautiful people were filled with life, even when life wasn't exactly easy living. These kids had been to hell and back, but their spirits never wavered. My absolute favorite part was the dining hall. The food was marvelous and I was able to sit with my friends and talk about absolute nonsense. Camp made me realize I don't need to feel normal, I just need to be my best self and accept that.

After attending camp, I was able to meet with a new doctor for my episodes. She identified them as Paroxysmal Dyskinesia, which is a muscular movement disorder that was likely caused by inflammation in the brain due to my tumor. She prescribed a seizure medication that has completely stopped the episodes. For a while I wasn't allowed to be very independent. I was afraid to cross the street by myself in fear of having an episode and getting hurt. Now that my episode are gone I regained my freedom and am not as self-conscious as before. My pediatrician has cleared me to get my driver's license and I am working on learning to drive. I am a straight A student, and I am also able to take and assist in karate classes again.

I haven't fully recovered, but I am doing so much better. There were days during recovery where I asked myself why I put myself through something so traumatic, but I realized I wanted to not only survive, but I wanted to live my life to its fullest potential. So I chose a year of recovery and surgery over a lifetime of unhappiness and pain. Bob Marley once said, "You never know how strong you are until being strong is your only choice." I had to be courageous and brave because being those things were the only chance I had at living an extraordinary life. Now that I have had brain surgery, there is nothing I can't do.

xoxo

GiGi

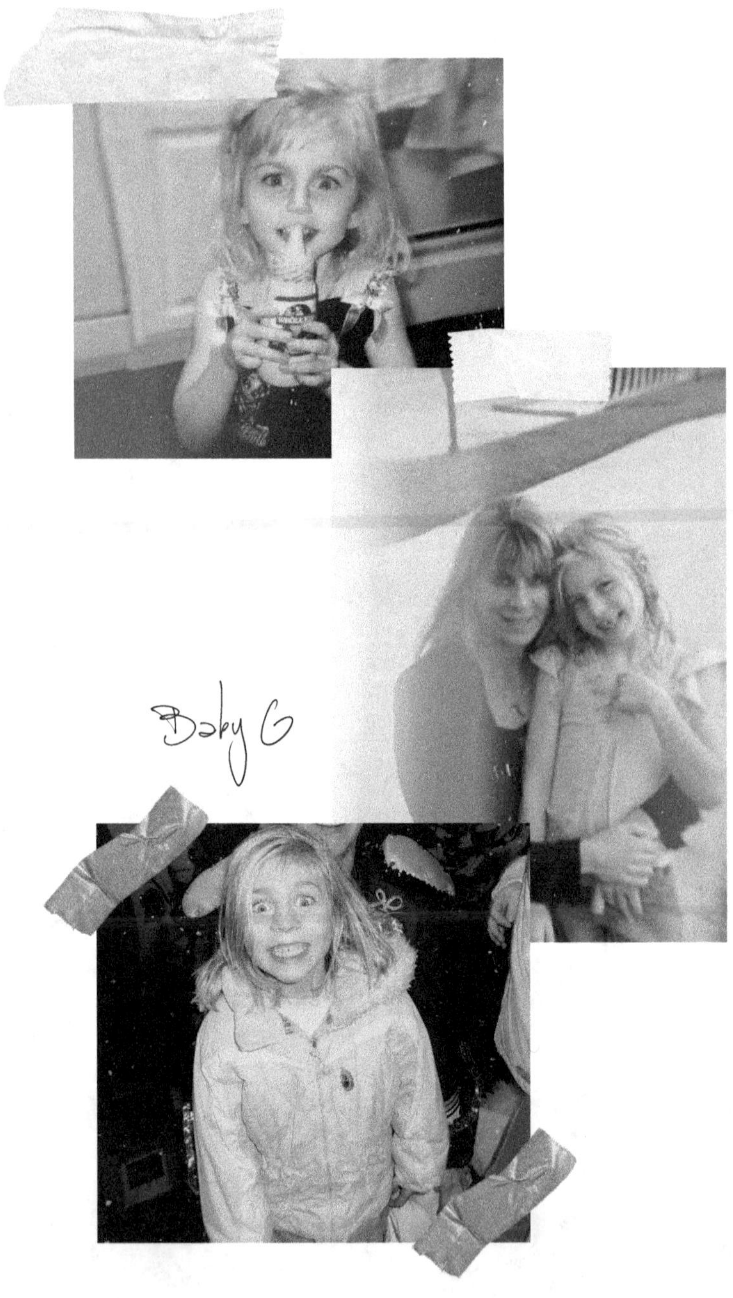
Baby G

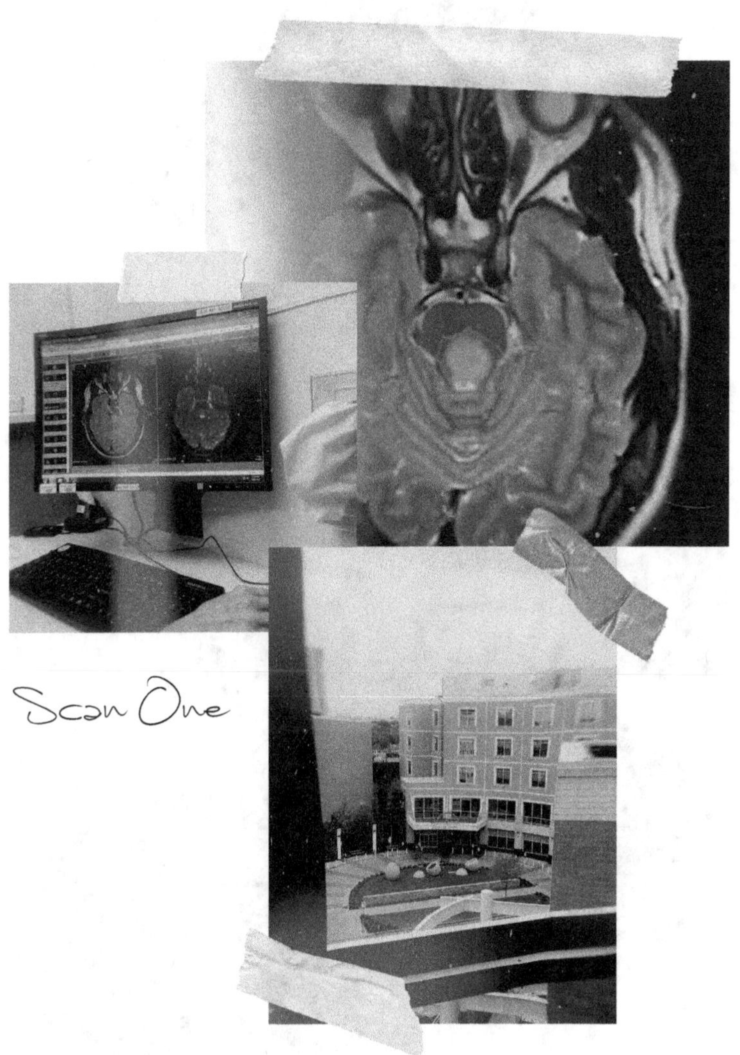

Scan One

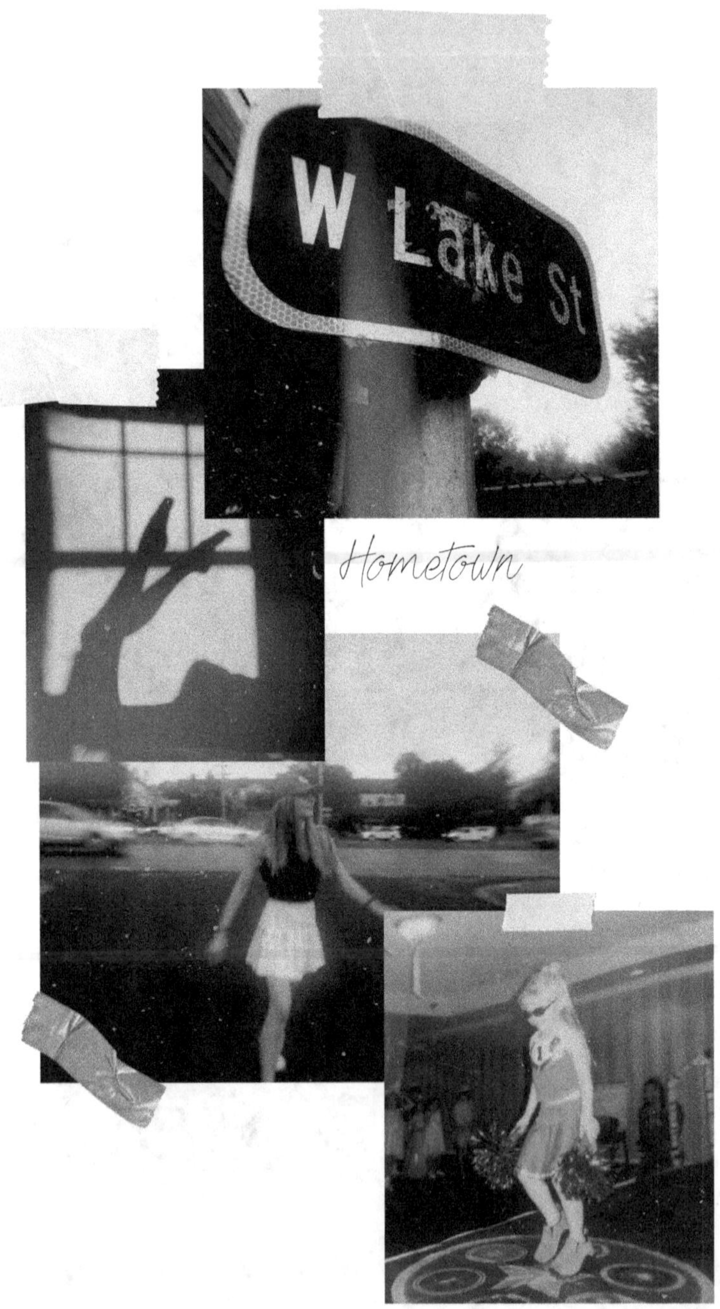
W Lake St
Hometown
5th Birthday

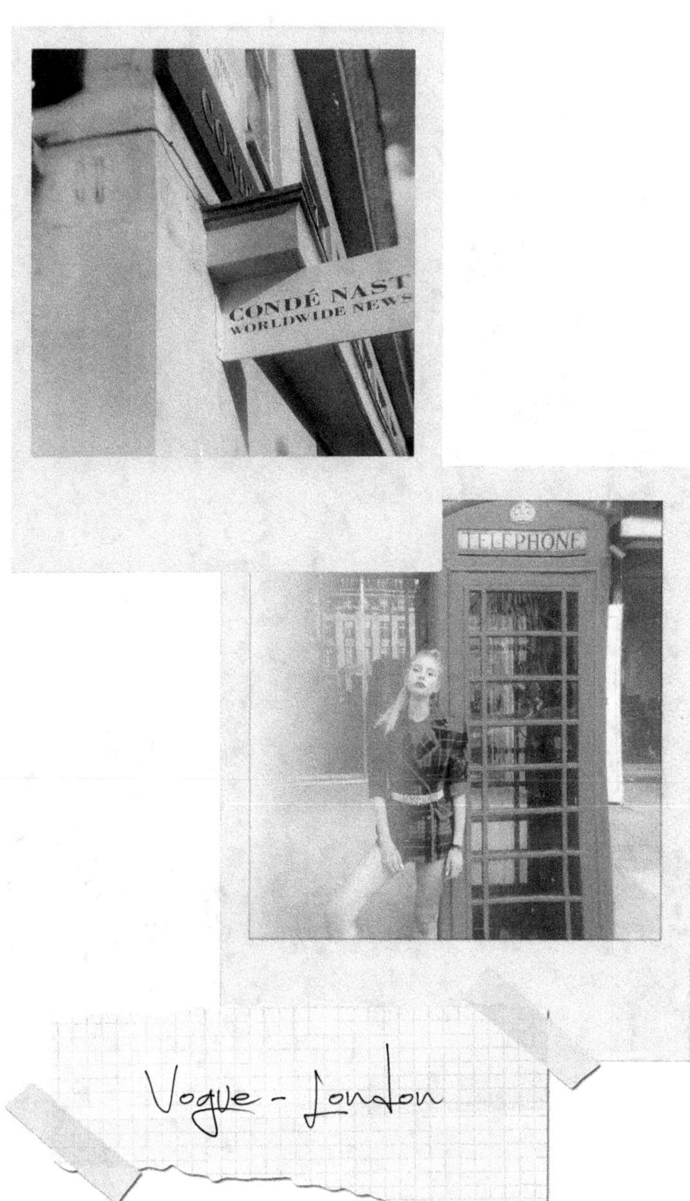
CONDÉ NAST
WORLDWIDE NEWS
TELEPHONE
Vogue - London

Beverly Hills, CA

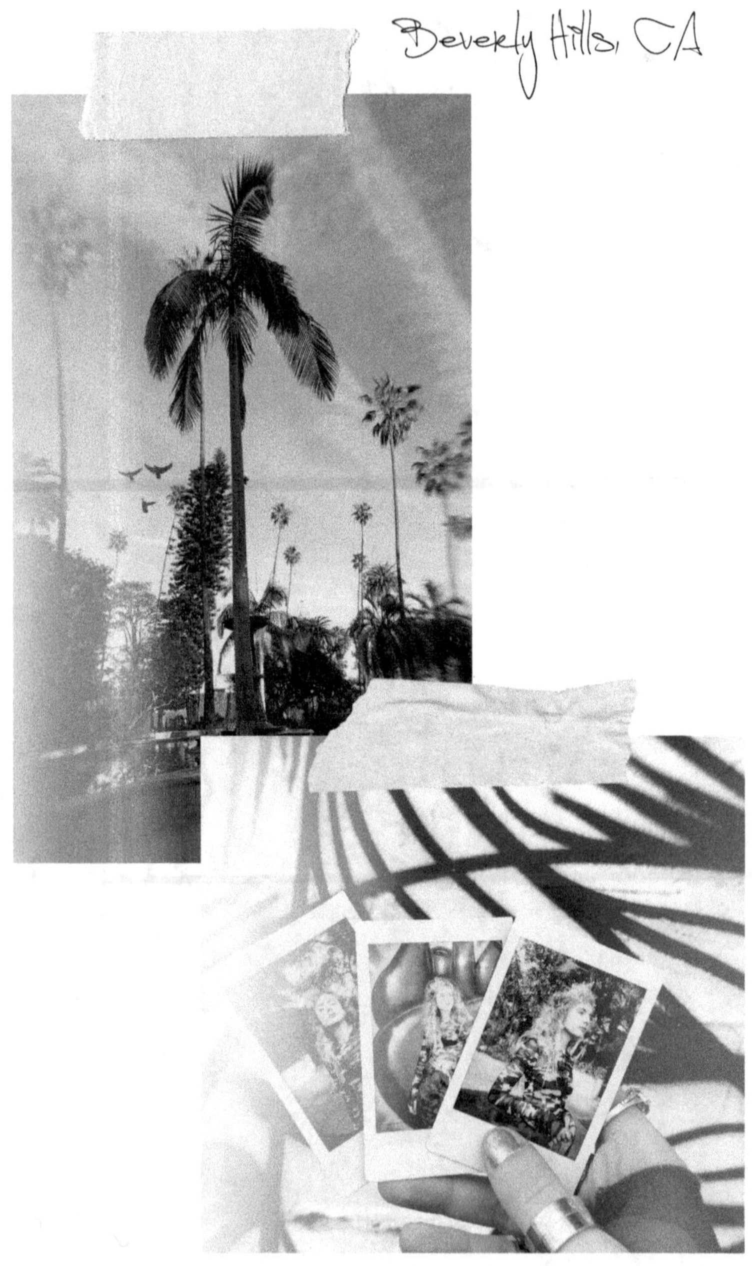

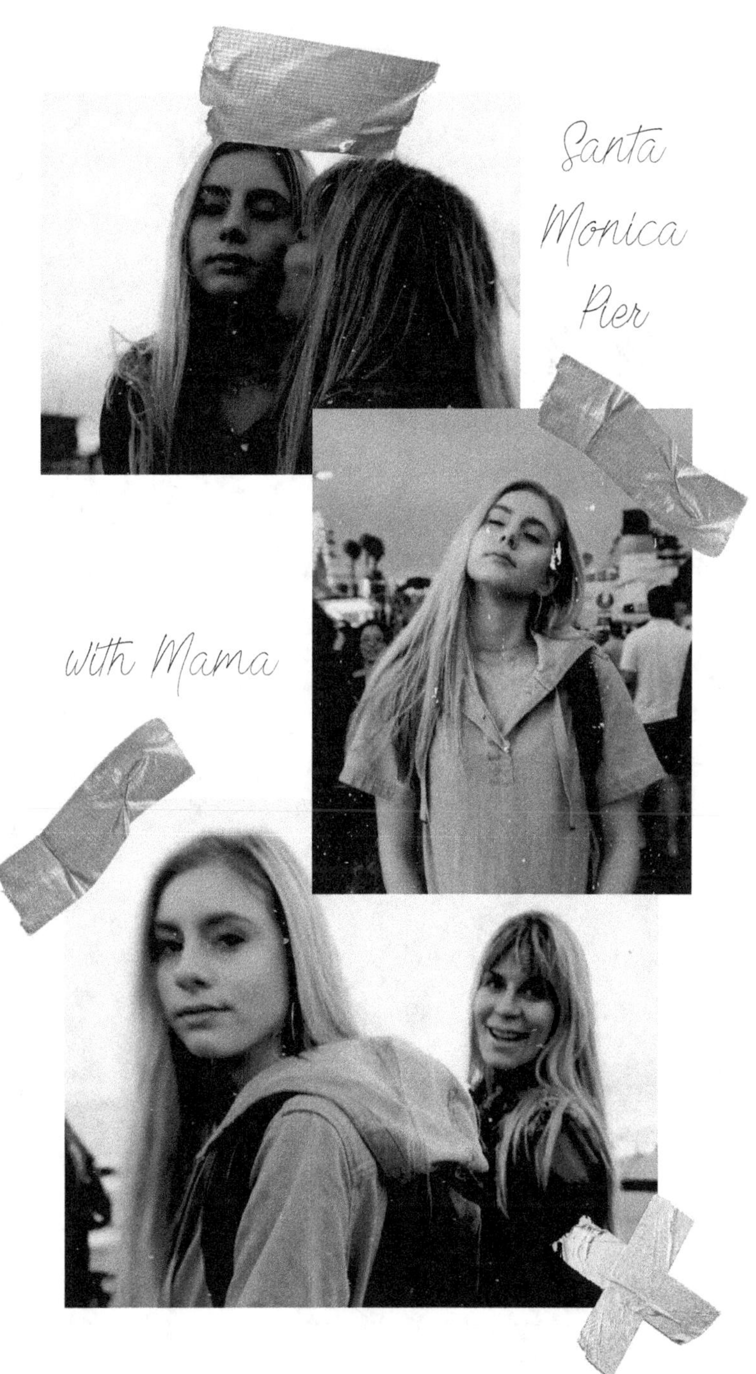
Santa
Monica
Pier

with Mama

UNDER

breath
she says
count down from 10
she says
i don't know why i listen
but i do

maybe
it's because her voice sounds gentle
or because
i can't bear to keep my eyes open anyways

in i breath
the scent of the peppermint chapstick inside
the mask fills my lungs

in i breath
slowly at first
but then all at once
the room turns
black

"You're So Lucky"

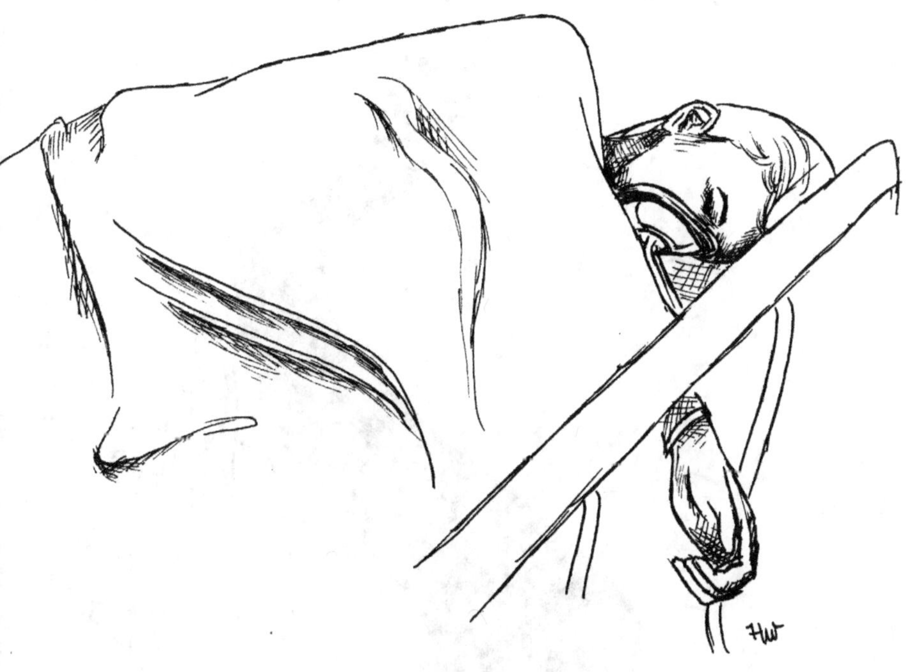

Sketch By Heather Rosati

Grace Ash Wethor

Sketch By Maryline Platevoet

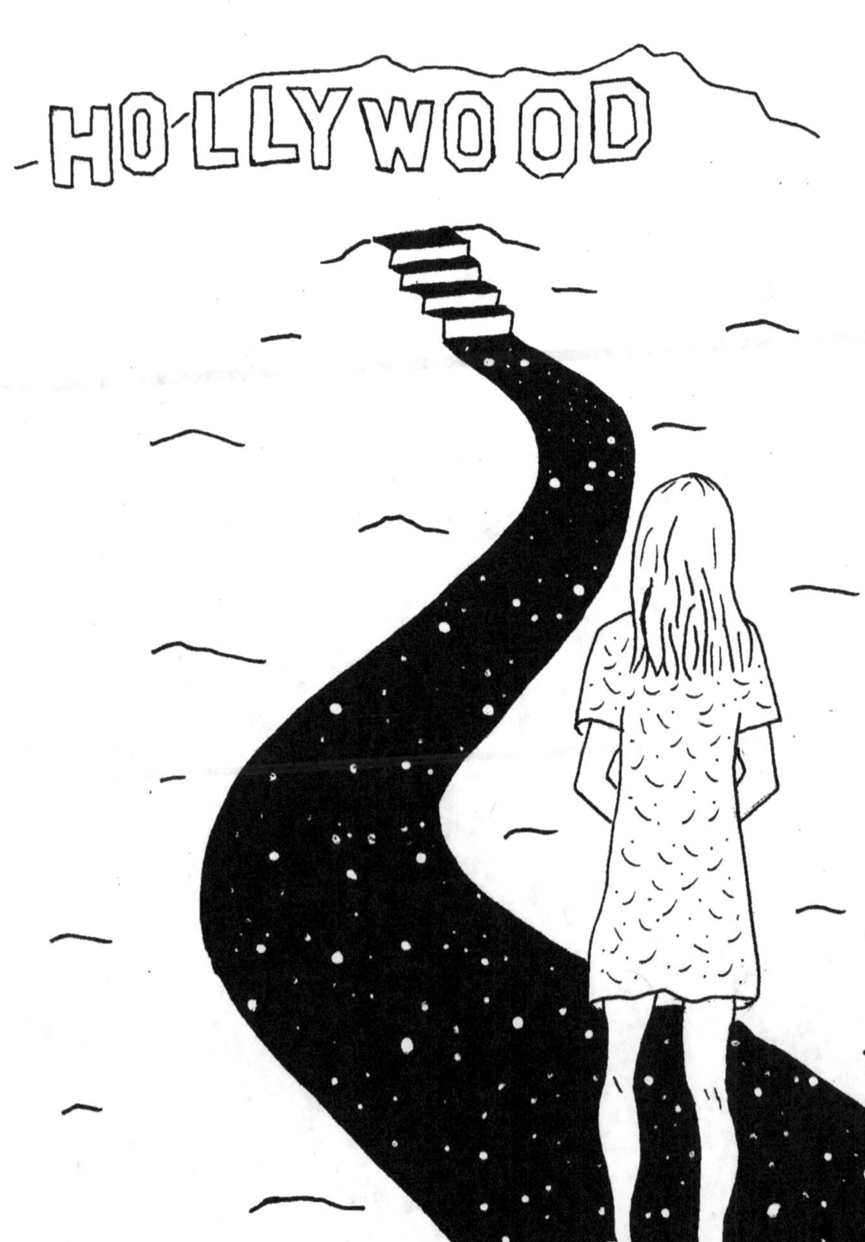

Hannah Montana

i remember being fascinated
with Hannah Montana when i was little

she was normal during the day
and then she would jet off
to movie premieres and red carpets

having a double life
a two faced mask
a place to escape and live her dreams
and become someone else

and then i did
i became her
there are two of me
sick me
HOLLYWOOD me

sometimes they occur individually
and sometimes they occur simultaneously
it depends on the day

one time I woke up
spent the day in the hospital
got on a plane
and walked in New York Fashion Week
that night

i am Hannah Montana
literally

NOT

I am not my tumor
I am not exhaustion
I am not headaches
I am not doctors visits
I am not medication
I am not MRIs
I am not an illness
I am strong
I am alive
I am a survivor
I will not stop dreaming
I will not stop hoping
I will not stop believing
I will move forward
because I am a survivor

"You're So Lucky"
Sketch By Maryline Platevoet

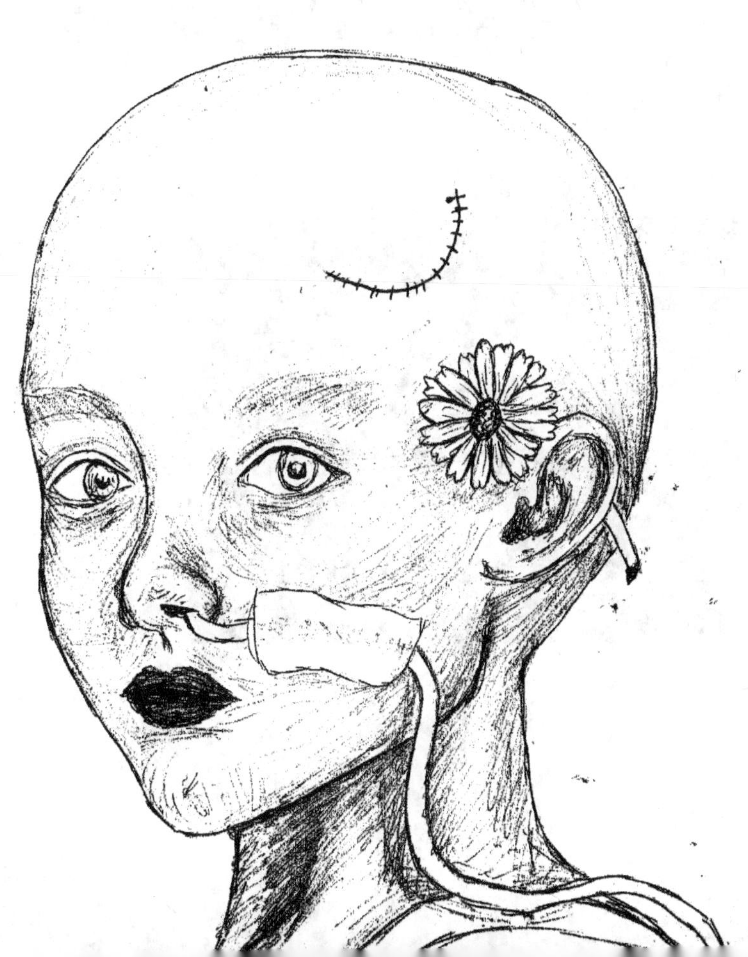

Ted Talk

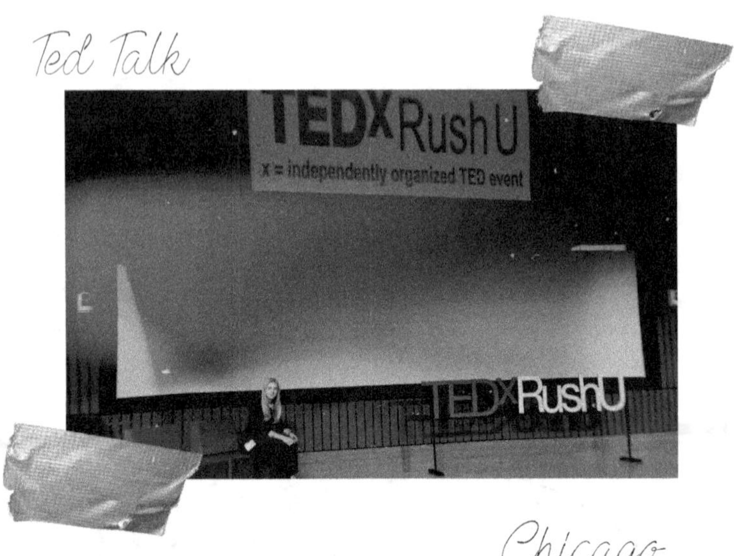

Chicago

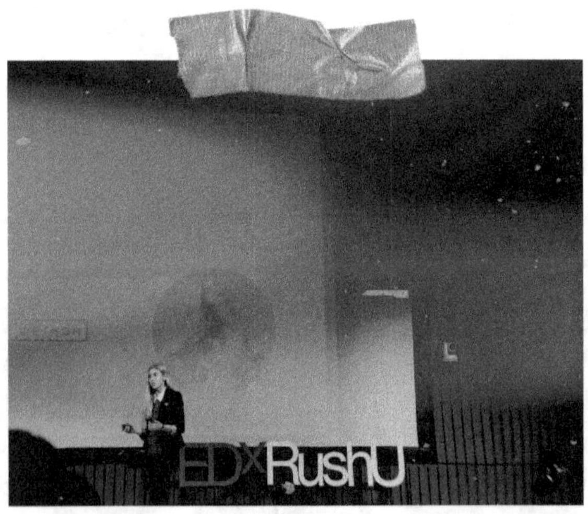

Dear TED,

I talked about my tumor when people asked, but I never REALLY talked about it. My Ted Talk was the first time I did. I grew up watching Ted Talks in class and quickly became fascinated with the idea of people sharing their experiences and their stories with the community. That's why when I was asked to give a Ted Talk of my own, I ran around my room screaming and crying for about three hours. I know that may seem excessive, but when you achieve something that you never really thought would ever be possible, you freak out a little.

 I found out two weeks before so I didn't have a very long time to prepare. Finally the day came and we headed off to Chicago. I lost my voice because I had been practicing so much and we missed our flight, so it was kind of a hectic day. However, everything turned out amazing and it was truly a life changing experience.

 That day was the first time I truly realized I wanted to share my story and hopefully reach others who had been going through similar things. So I guess you could thank TED for this whole book…

Thank you to everyone who made that day possible.

With Love,

J

Alexa Ponciano

Ependymomas Tumor Survivor

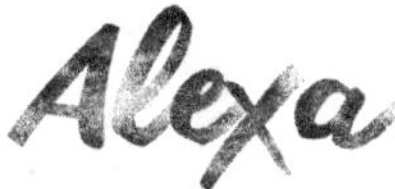

Imagine being 10 years old, going to birthday parties and not being able to eat all the goodies like the cakes, cupcakes or pizza. Or imagine getting severe headaches every night for months and nothing helping the pain. That was me as a kid, and here's my story.

When I was about 6 years old I started getting severe stomach pains, it was constant and they wouldn't stop. Every night I would cry to my parents about how bad they were. It was the same routine, go to school, come home, get stomach pains and headaches and feel so bad. As we were trying to figure out the problem, I remember everyone trying to figure out what was going on. Maybe she's lactose intolerant, maybe she's making it up, maybe she's stressed at school. And all I would say is fix me! At that point I didn't care what was wrong I just wanted the pain to go away.

After six months of constant pains and tons of doctors' visits, my family had enough of it and we were done being in the dark. We pushed hard to see what was wrong, and thanks to my mom she pushed for a blood test which revealed I had celiac disease.

Celiac disease is a serious autoimmune disease where your immune system responds by damaging the finger-like villi of the small intestine. The pain can be brought on by some of your favorite foods and snacks including bread, cakes, brownies, pizza, pasta, chicken nuggets and much more. All my favorite foods at 6 years old were problems for me.

It was a difficult time for me, because 9 years ago people didn't understand celiac disease as well as they do now, and I felt as though I had nothing to eat. All the fun foods were off limits. I went to parties and had to bring my own pizza and cupcakes which I thought was embarrassing, I was that kid. To me at that age it was frustrating because I was left out of the joys of eating my favorite food and being like any other kid my age. I just wanted to fit in. To this day it is hard still to tell people I don't want that cookie, brownie, pizza because if I eat it I'll suffer the consequences. Today people bring gluten free food and I can eat the things I enjoy. And the one benefit is now I can encourage others that if they are feeling pain they should go to the doctor and push for that simple blood test.

As I solved one problem another occurred. My headaches were becoming more severe and I was just starting my new diet, we thought maybe it was my body trying to adjust to the changes or that I was still eating things that had gluten.

We went back to the doctors and were referred to a neurologist. We were in there for a good hour going over family history, my life at home, at school and just trying to figure out why these headaches were so severe. Again, I had the same feeling as before, I just want to be a normal kid and solve the problem. I had enough of all the pain.

At the end of my appointment the doctor turned to my mom and said he believed that I was suffering from migraines and he wanted to put me on migraine medicine. I was 8 years old and this doctor wanted to put me on medicine. My mom immediately said no, she explained that I was just diagnosed with celiac and was afraid that maybe we were missing something in my diet. She believed we would be masking the problem. I clearly remember the doctor not being happy and said to her, and his exact words, "fine, I'll order up a cat scan but I can bet my career on it we won't find anything." I remember over the years my mom telling this story to family, friends, strangers that as she left the doctor's office with the phone number in hand, she thought to herself, should she call and make an appointment for that CT scan. She tells people that she kept saying to herself, he's the doctor, he would know and after all he is betting his career on it that nothing is wrong. She later told me she had this gut feeling that she shouldn't listen to the doctor and that she needed to follow her mother's instinct. And that is what she did and she made that appointment.

My mom reminds me that she took me into the office for my CT scan and everything seemed normal. She never felt as though brain tumor would ever come out of anyone's mouth about me. The next day she got a call while she was at work from my dad, he was crying uncontrollably and said he needed to talk to her. My mom said that she remembers asking him if it was about his mom, his dad, his siblings. And my dad said no. He said you just need to get to my office immediately. She tells everyone that she remembers every part of that day like it was yesterday. She remembers that it was pouring, windy and storming that day and she was driving extra careful but as she was on her way she said to herself, I asked him about everyone but the kids. She was so mad at herself for not asking about us. When she got to my dad's office she remembers that he was sitting at a big conference table and he was balling his eyes out. He had just gotten a call from the neurologist and that they had discovered that I indeed had a brain tumor.

My parents waited for the doctors to call them back to explain what was going on with me. When the phone rang and they answered it they were unsure of what was going to be said. His first words to them was an apology. He apologized for the comments he made to my mom, about betting his career on not finding a tumor. He said in all his career he never had seen a case where the only symptoms were headaches. At that point it wasn't even worth arguing with him about. It was about finding out what the next steps were to make sure I was going to survive and be healthy.

The doctor explained that the tumor was sitting on the cerebellum into the spinal column. Two days after my CT scan I was admitted into Stanford Hospital to go through a battery of tests. I had endless MRIs that weekend and I was poked and prodded multiple times, as a little kid I was deathly afraid of needles. It was not something I allowed to happen easily. The night before my surgery the nurses came in and informed us that they were going to shave parts of my head. I was so upset about it and knew that this was going to make me look so different. Not only was I not able to eat normal foods like the other kids, but I have a brain tumor and my head was going to be shaved.

The next morning, President's Day, I went in for my 8-hour surgery, successfully removing the tumor. My goal after surgery was getting out of the hospital and going to my own home and bed. Recovery seemed easy for me, maybe because I was so young. I slept a lot and made sure that if I wasn't sleeping I was resting and not over doing it. My parents were right there by my side the whole time. I did miss a lot of school but that was fine with me!

One afternoon I wanted to, no I needed to, get out of the house so I went with my mom to pick up my twin brother from school. I guess I thought no big deal, I'm here with parts of my head shaved, I just had major brain surgery, I'll be ok. Well it wasn't the pain of the scar, or where they removed my tumor, it was the pain of being bullied. I was bullied by one girl.

This girl was with her mother across the yard from where we were and yelled across the way how ugly I looked, pointed at me, laughed at me and just made fun of how different I looked from others. It was heartbreaking for me.

As a young kid who was dealing with all these issues now had someone who hated me and wanted to bully me because she didn't feel good about herself. And her mother was just as bad because she didn't say anything to her child. It was a difficult time but with the help of my family and real friends I got through it. When I went through surgery, I realized that people go through things and even though they don't have a right to be hateful, you need to tell yourself that you don't care about the comments and remember that no matter what the circumstances are, you are beautiful and no one can say anything differently.

When you are dealing with health problem in your life, you don't want people to feel bad for you or change the way they treat you. As for me, I wanted people to treat me the same as they would if none of this had ever happened, be supportive and be my friend. Now when I see someone bald walking down the street or somebody with a birth defect I don't want to point it out or label them differently, I want to think of them as a strong individual, a beautiful person who is trying to make the most out of the beautiful life they have. People might not show their feelings of fear or sadness to others but going through what I did, I know that there are those feelings so don't judge others or be rude to them because you never know what they are going through in their life or the struggles they are dealing with. Be nice to everybody, share a smile, say hi, open doors for them. I want others to know that there are still compassionate people in the world. Your kindness can truly help someone get through the day.

I love spending time with my family, especially my mom, and my best friends. Surrounding myself with the people I love empowers me to do anything, because of them I have courage and confidence and love doing new things. I love adventure and have learned to take advantage of right now. I always say to myself, "never regret anything because it makes you a stronger person and do things you love in the moment because you may never be able to experience that love again."

One thing my mom my and I both believe is to always be an advocate for yourself. If you aren't feeling well, you get in to the doctors and make sure they find out what is wrong. Don't let someone say to you that they will bet their career they won't find anything. You know your body and you know you aren't the same.
Fight and never give up!

My life has forever been changed but I hope that my experiences can help those that are facing the unknown and to let them know they are not alone and there are still people in this world who truly care. Brain tumors can't stop you from living your life and being happy.

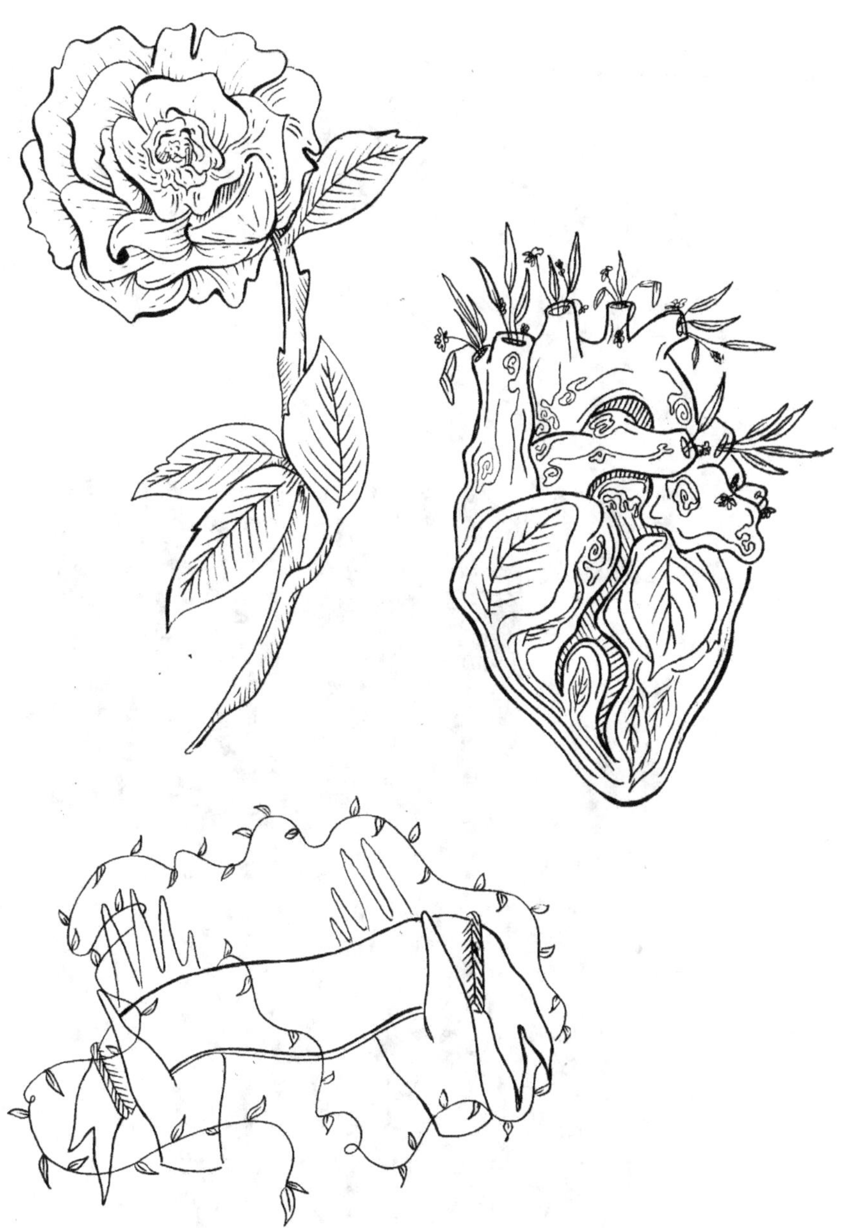

Sketch By Jaiden Bjorklund

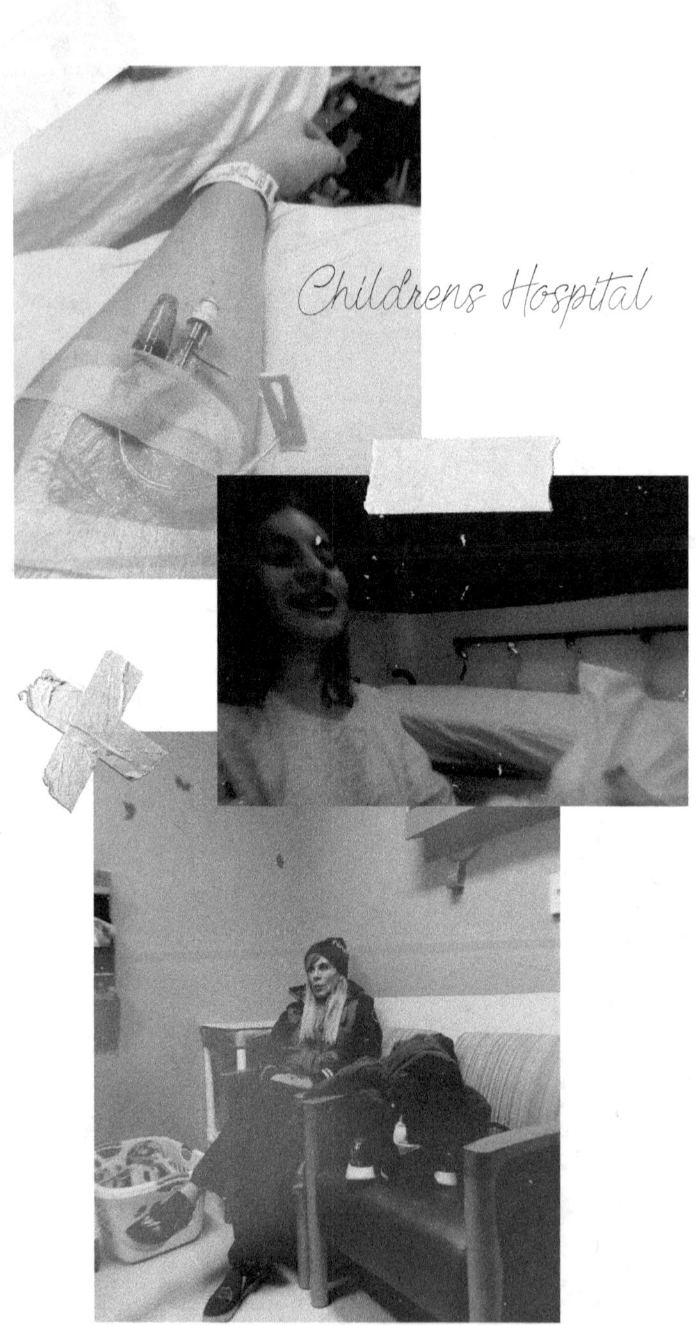

Childrens Hospital
Minneapolis, MN

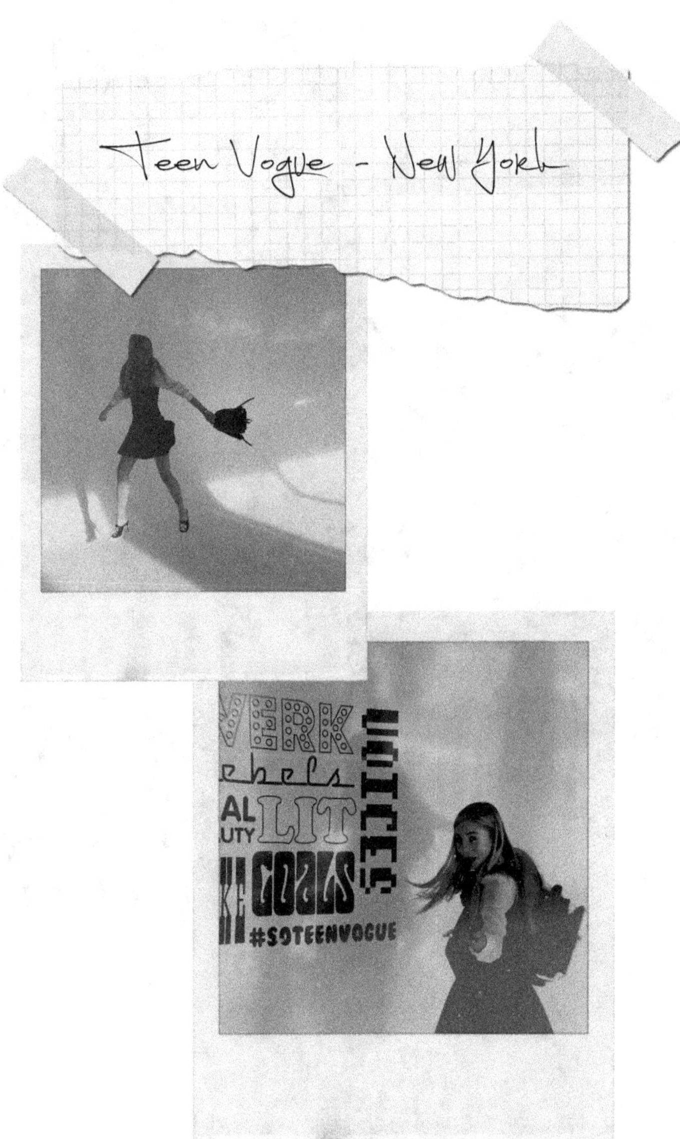

Teen Vogue - New York

YERK
ebels
AL LIT
UTY
GOALS
#SOTEENVOGUE

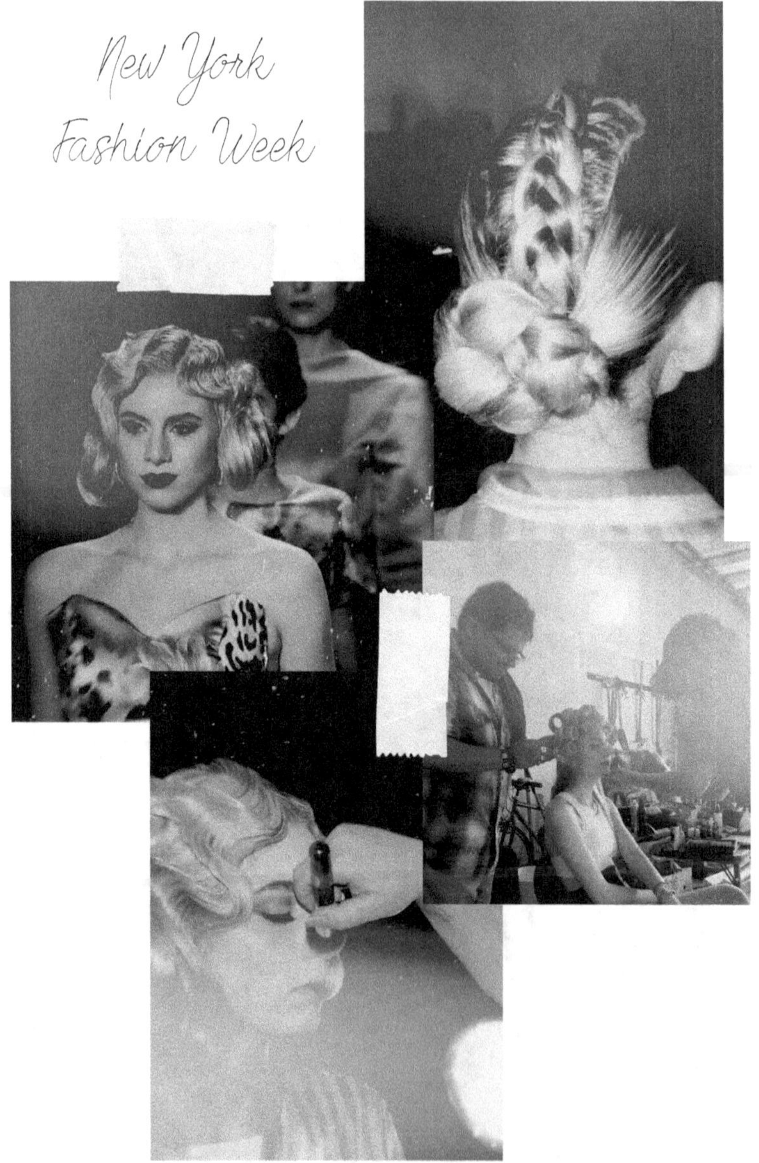
New York
Fashion Week

PressPlay

Orange County, CA

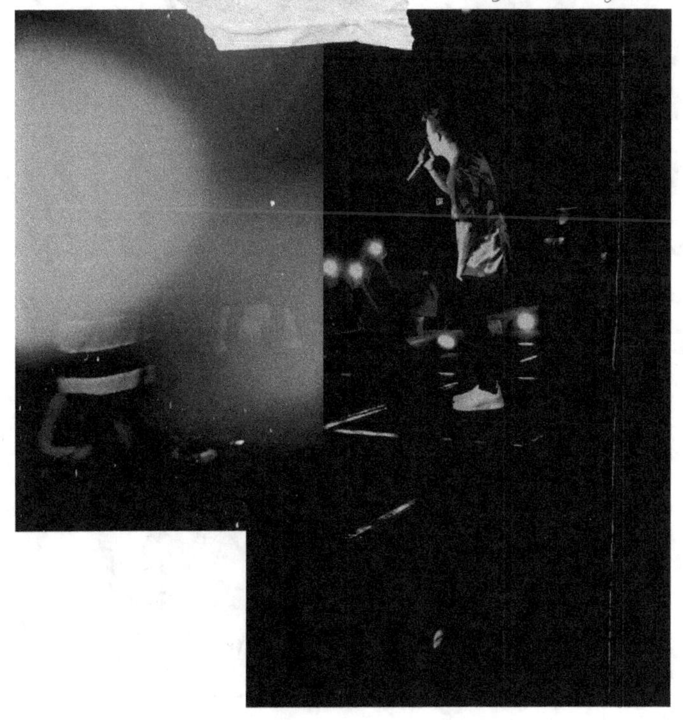

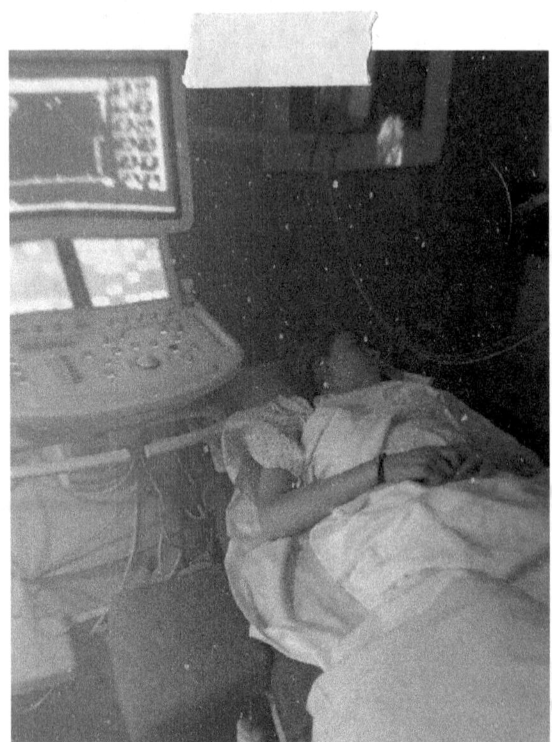

Mayo Clinic

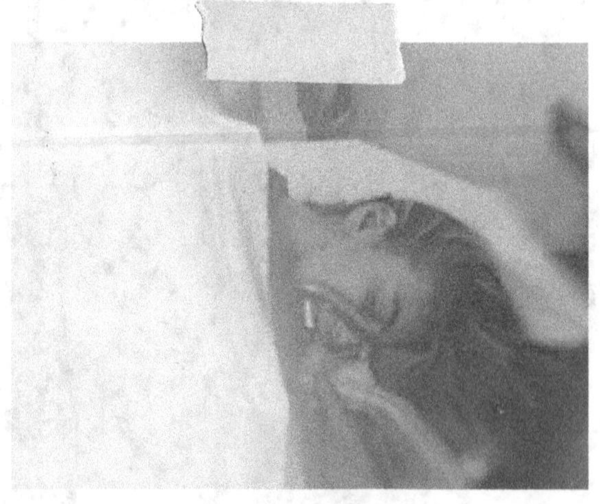

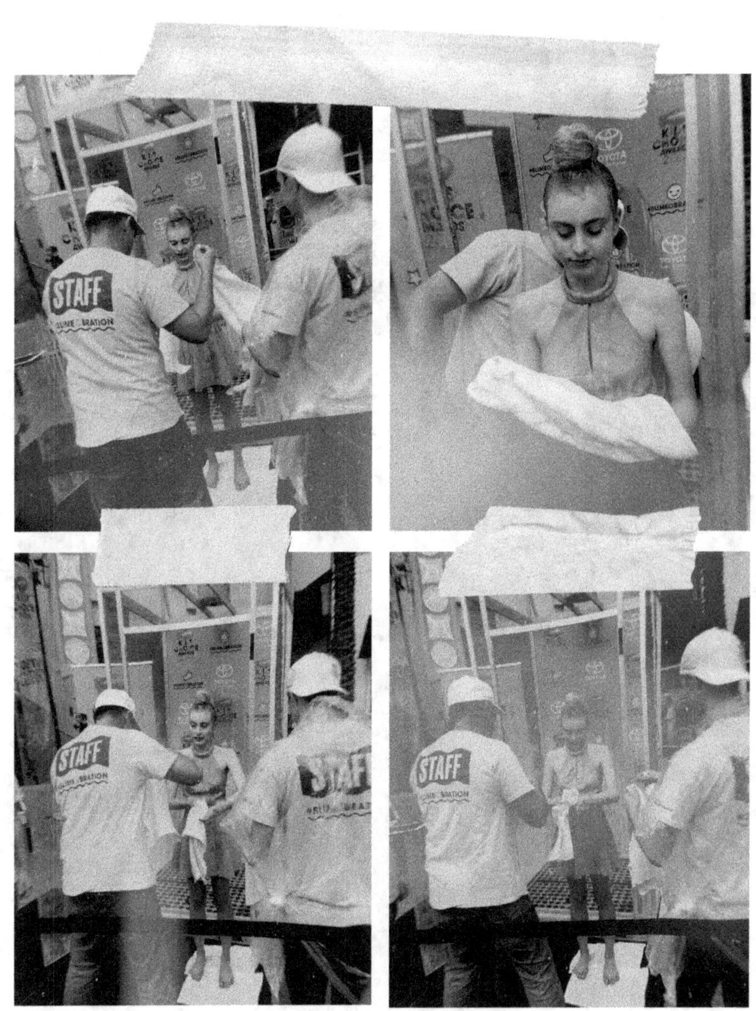

Nickelodeon
Kids Choice Awards

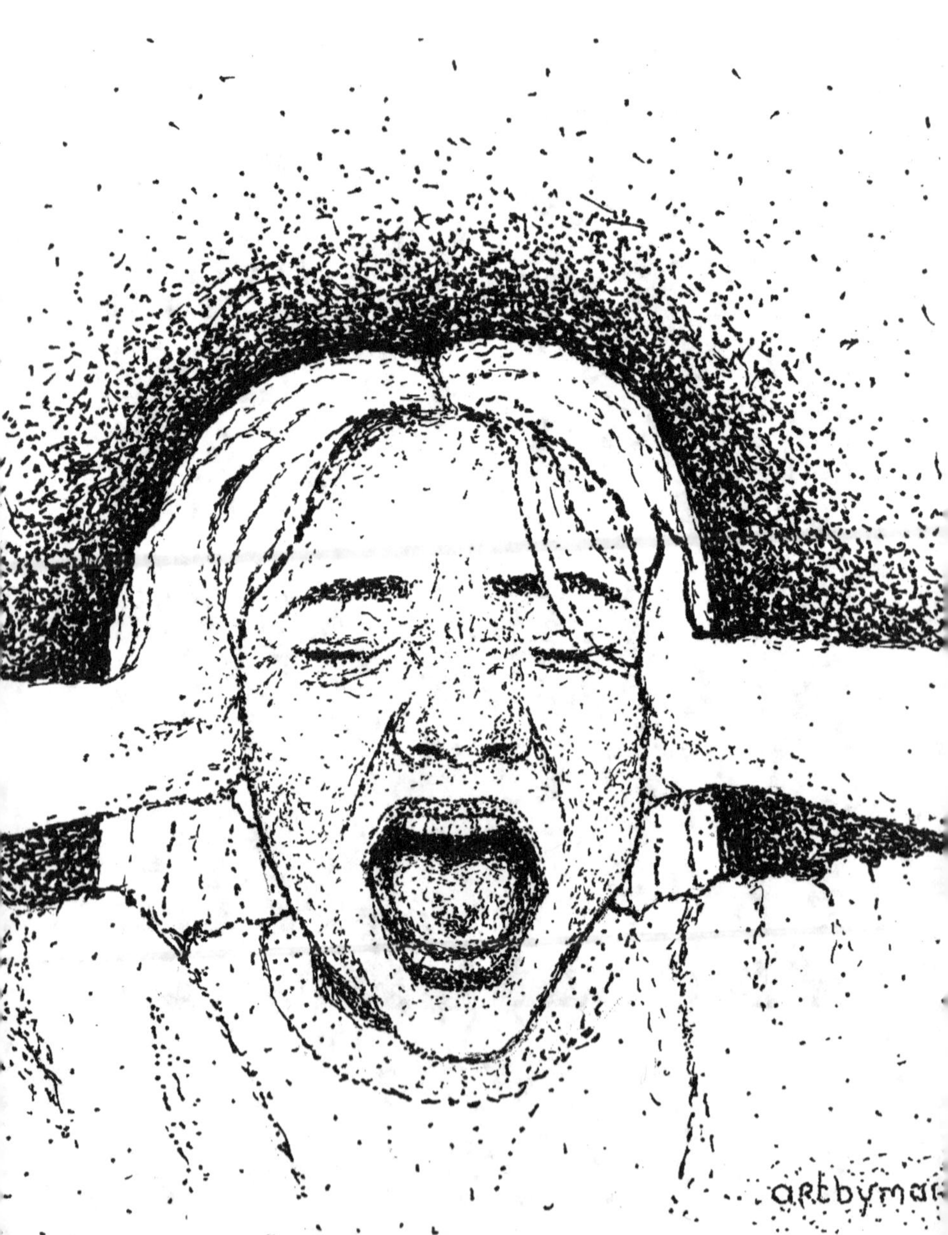

Sketch By Maryline Platevoet

SCREAM

i love horror books
but i hate horror movies
IDK
it's this weird in-between
when ideas
turn to images
to reality

it's kind of like an illness
when it turns from something
on tv
in the news
trending on twitter

into your reality...

PLASTIC

they think they know us
they don't know
what goes on behind this show
what goes on behind this glow
what goes on behind this bow

plastic manufactured lives
playing with their plastic knives
do they even think we cry
when we see their hate online…

i could be barbie
you could be ken
no emotions til' the end
did they think when they hit send
guess we'll just have to unfriend

they think their lives are real great
plastic words shoved in they brains
by housewives
they're all the same
even they call the kids names

to my face you call me lame
cause your friends all think the same
but last week you called me called me great
are you really sure
I'm the one who is fake?

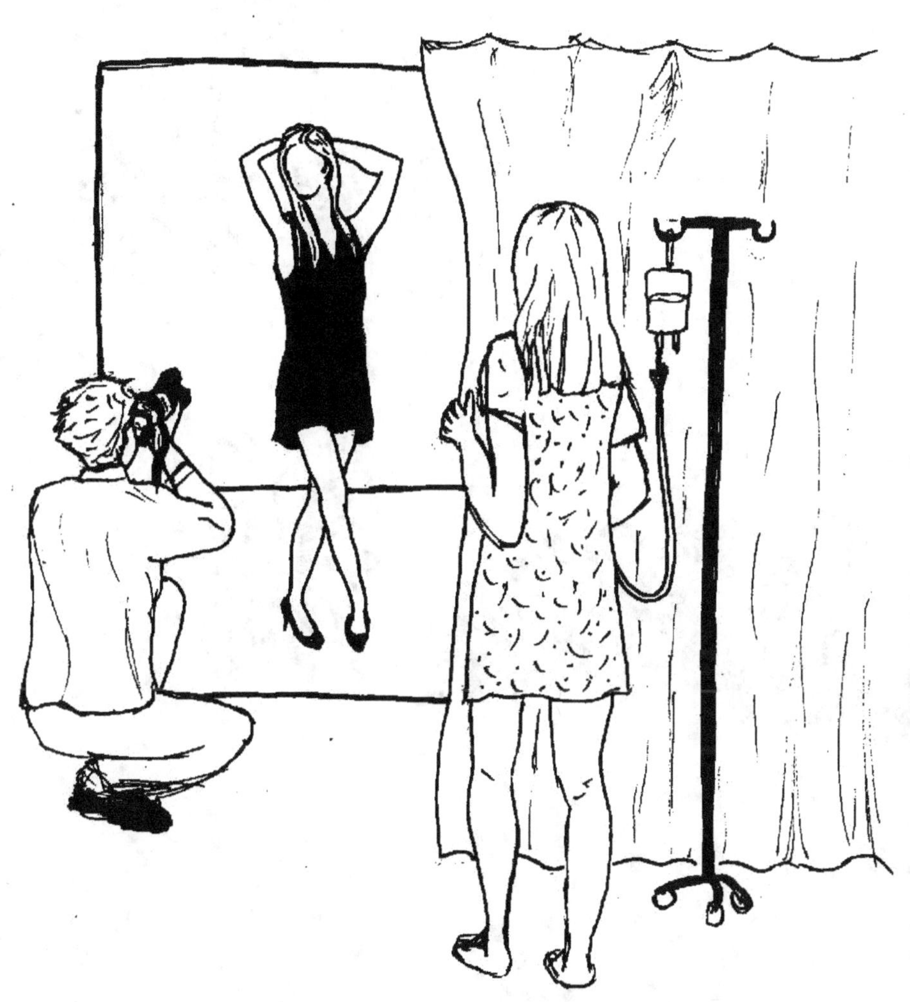

Sketch By Maryline Platevoet

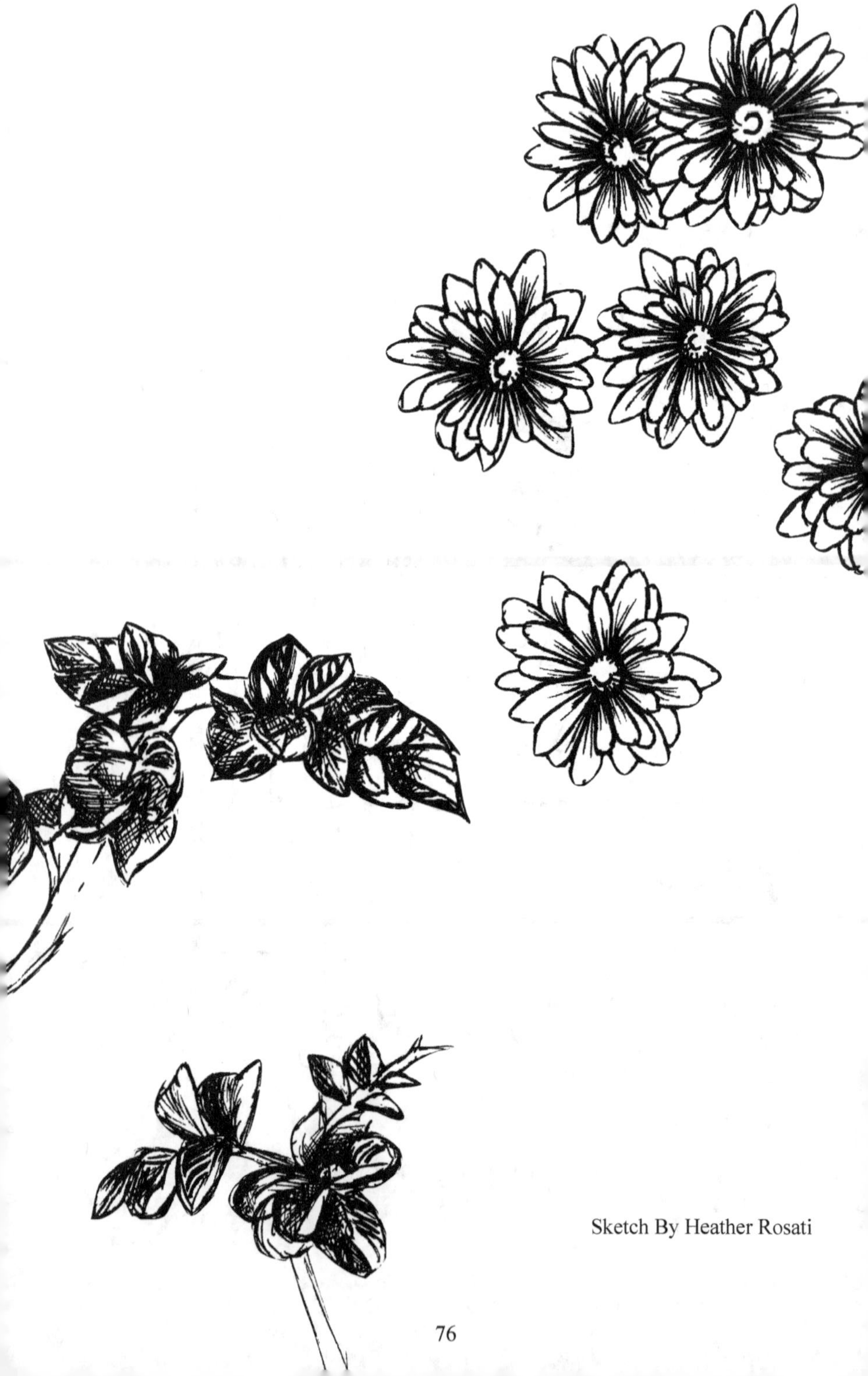

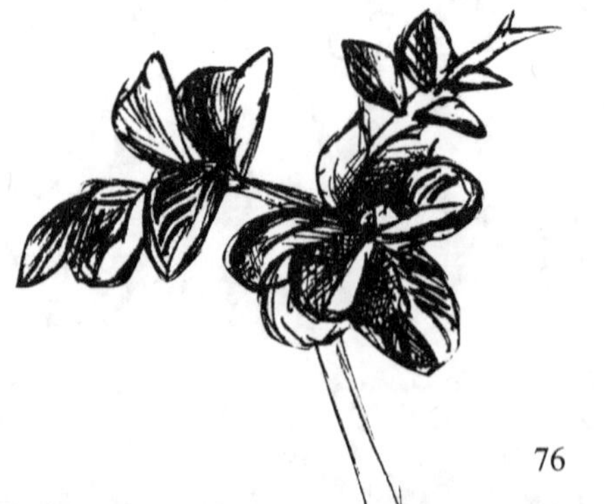

Sketch By Heather Rosati

Gathering Grounds

remember when we
slurped raspberry lime smoothies...

in that weird corner
of that weird restaurant
in that weird town in
northern Minnesota

we had adventures back then...

in that weird cabin
with the weird backyard
on that weird lake

it seems so distant
like it never actually happened...

did it?

was that swaying apple tree ripe
was that run down grocery store solid brick
was that dusty antique store authentic
were those iced raspberry smoothies
nothing but a figment of my imagination...

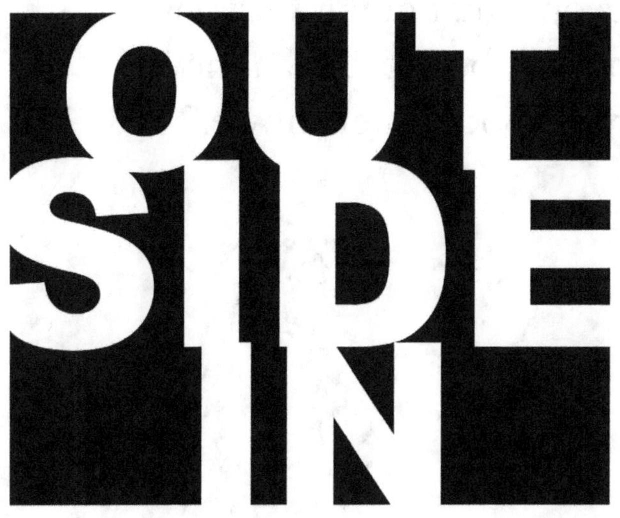

My Cancer Journey
3 Years Later,
**From The Minds Of Those Who
Lived It.**

"She used this opportunity to
show people that going for your
dreams can be more than the
plot to a good disney movie."

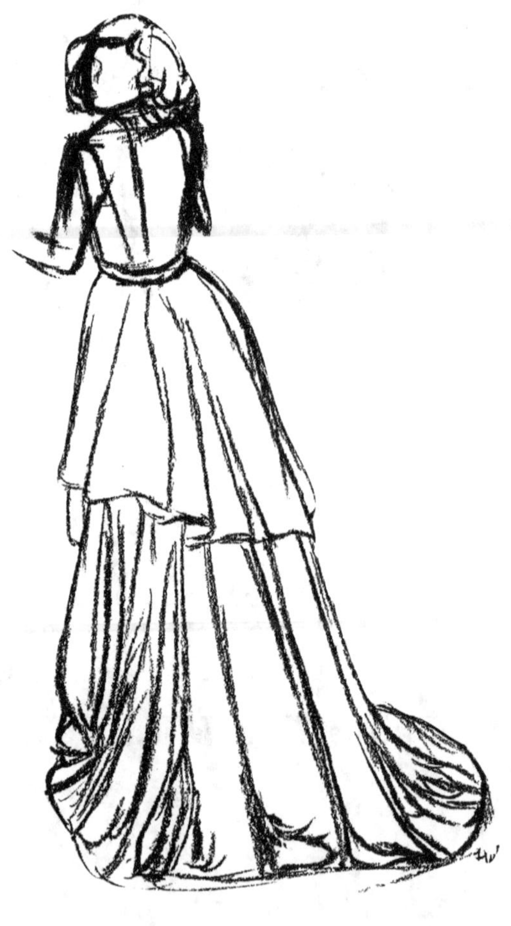

Sketch By Heather Rosati

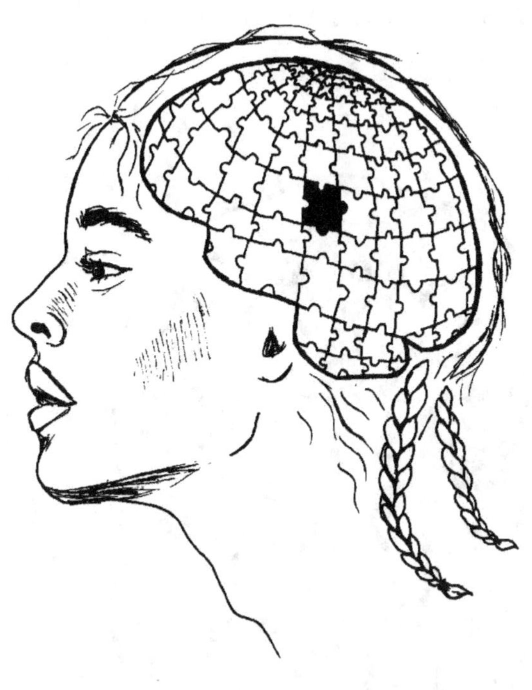

"She walked into gym class; her eyes were purple and yellow. You could tell she had been through a lot and something was wrong."

Sketch By Maryline Platevoet

"I remember thinking it was a joke,
but it wasn't.

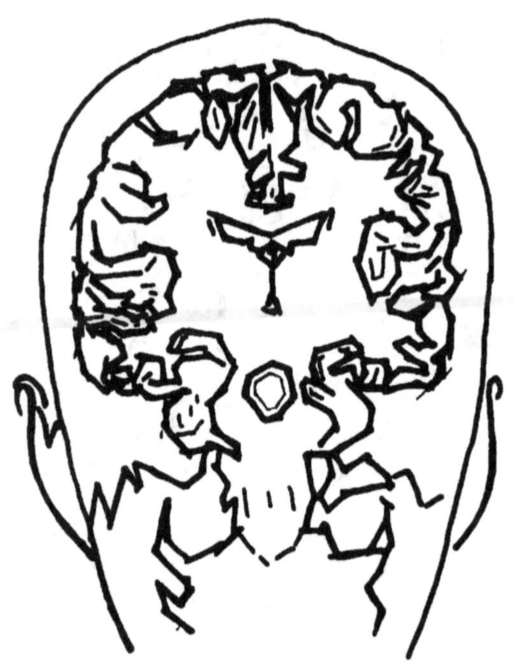

"I went home and I tried to be
superman. I wanted to start funds and
find a cure."

Sketch By Heather Rosati

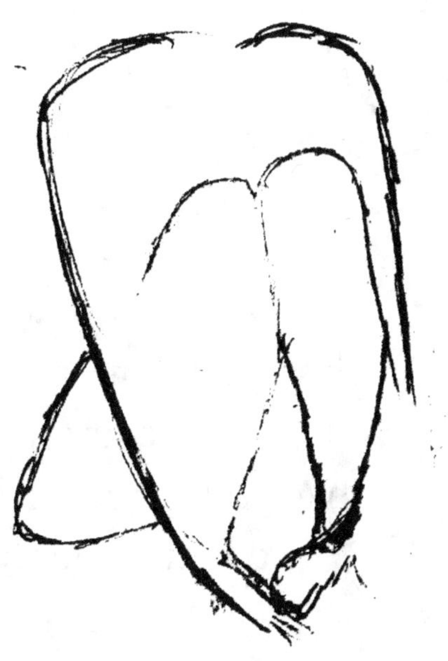

"Your mom told me, and showed me the photos. All I remember is being worried for you"

Sketch By Rachel Kramer

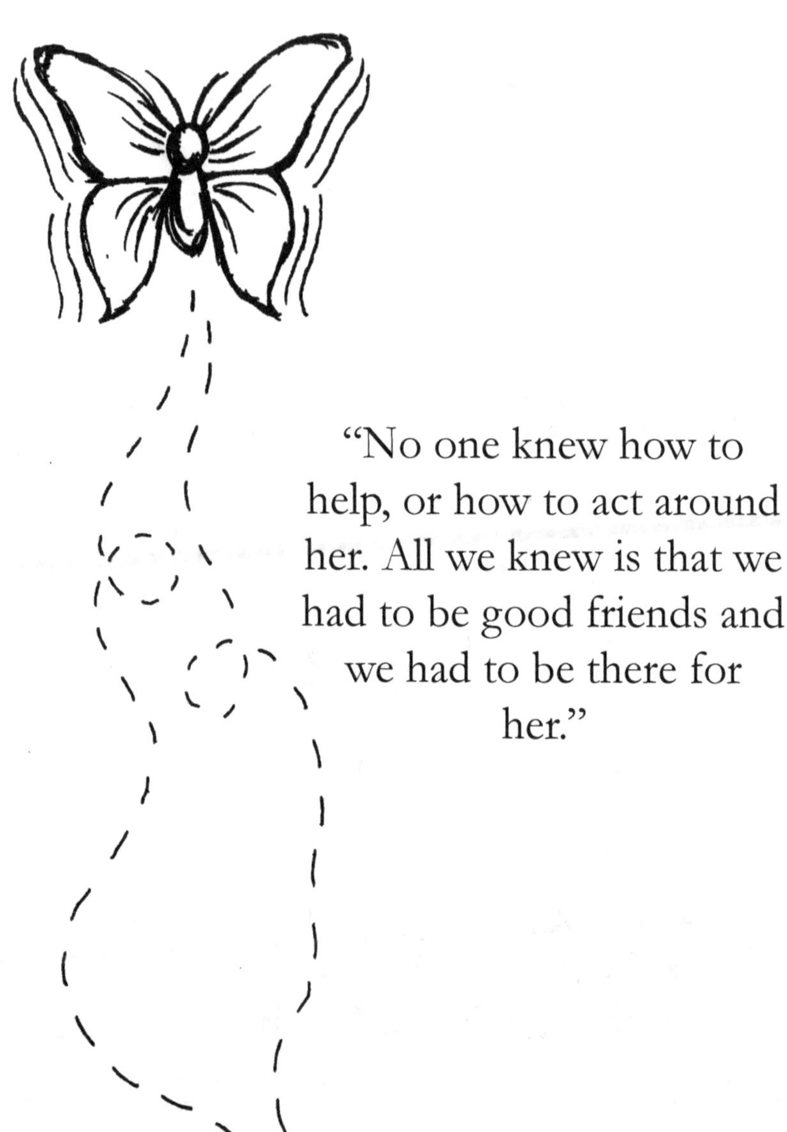

"No one knew how to help, or how to act around her. All we knew is that we had to be good friends and we had to be there for her."

Sketch By Heather Rosati

"I always thought of cancer being shown through hair loss or having to be in the hospital. But now I see it's all about perseverance.

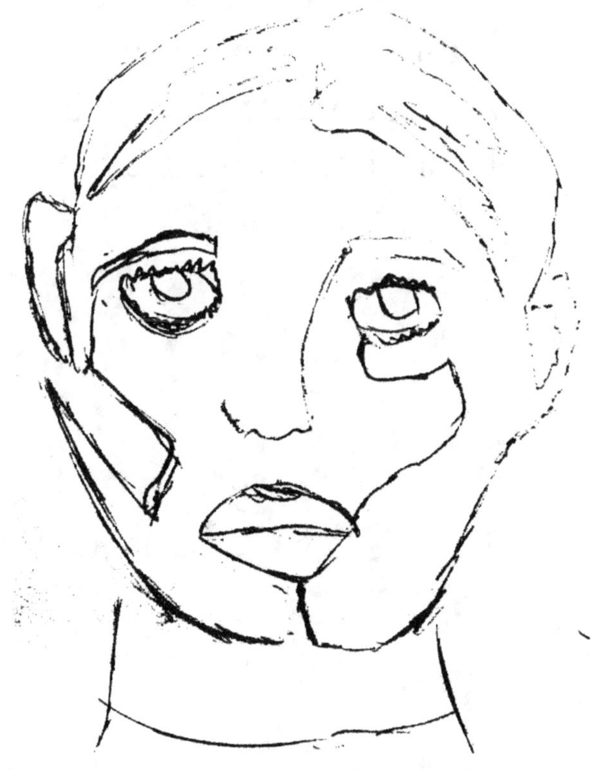

Sketch By Rachel Kramer

"She knew she wasn't going to be the girl who was diagnosed with a brain tumor and didn't live to tell about it."

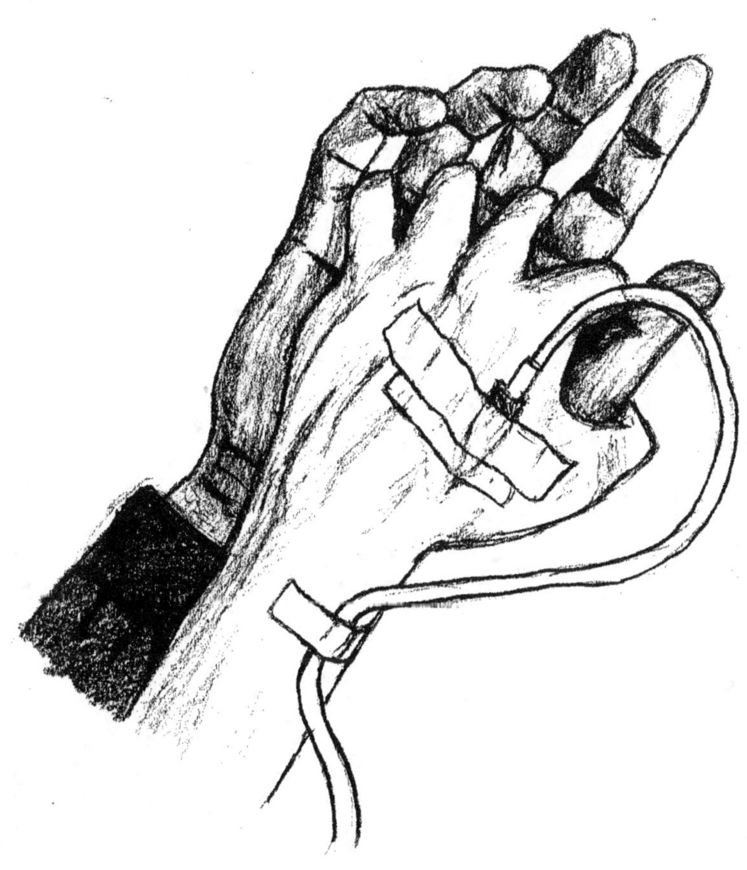

Sketch By Maryline Platevoet

Sierra Barnes

Craniopharyngioma Survivor

Featuring Sierra's Original Poetry and Paintings

Sierra

My name is Sierra Barnes. I'm 21 years old. I'm from Dallas, Texas. My journey started on December 20, 1996, the day I was born.

Everything seemed normal I was a healthy baby girl. As the years went on my Mom started to notice something wasn't quite right. We went to several doctors and they just couldn't seem to figure out what was going on. They would say things like I was eating too much and needed to be on a diet because of my weight. I was hardly eating so my Mom knew this wasn't the case.

In 2002 I was in a pageant. I had a terrible headache and didn't feel well the whole time. But I faked a smile through it anyway. My Mom thought I was just having a really bad sinus infection. The final day of the pageant, we went home that night. My head was still hurting really bad. My Mom asked if I needed to go to the hospital. I replied no because of course, no kid wants to go to the hospital. We laid there in my parents' bed and my mom happened to look over at me. I was clinching my forehead really tight because of all the pain. It was in that moment she knew we needed to go to the hospital.

It was that night that our lives would change forever. At the hospital, they did a CT scan that revealed I had a brain tumor. Later on, we found out it was Craniopharyngioma. When they told me I was going to have surgery I remember feeling angry and scared. I stormed around in the room with anger and tears. I told my Mom **"you just brought me here to die."** Which I don't think now but I said it out of fear and anger. Of course, these words broke my mom's heart to hear her daughter speak.

It was nine days later that I had surgery to remove it. Everything went great with the surgery. The doctor told my parents I probably wouldn't communicate for a few weeks. But I proved them wrong and I was back to acting like a diva not long after being taken to recovery.

One of the difficulties I faced after surgery was having a severe allergic reaction to morphine. I was having severe hallucinations where I was seeing things that I feared the most such as clowns, the room was flooding, and at one point I was convinced my mom's face was bleeding. This was a very scary time for me. It lasted for about three days.

I got to come home from the hospital in October 2002. The following year I received radiation. Since then my tumor has remained stable and it even showed shrinkage on my last M.R.I. I also have a cyst on my optic nerve which also has shown shrinkage. In 2003, I received my wish from the Make A Wish Foundation Of North Texas to meet Actress/Singer Hilary Duff. It was a really fun and memorable time for me and my family. Everyone was so nice and great, including Hilary.

My tumor also causes other health issues such as panhypopituitarism, non-alcoholic cirrhosis of the liver, osteopenia, growth hormone deficiency, and weight gain. I've dealt with and overcame many obstacles and challenges due to my tumor and other things, and I still do today. I've also had other things such as being judged on my appearance throughout the years since I was very young. I just want for people to get to know me for me and not judge me on my looks or because I have a brain tumor.

One of the ways I've overcome many of these things is by creating art and writing poetry. After having my surgery and coming home from the hospital in 2002, my mom gave me a small canvas to paint on which would be one of my first paintings. I named it Complicated. At just the age of five years old I was expressing my thoughts and feelings through art. I don't think I really even knew what art was or how it would help me. I just knew it was something that I really enjoyed doing.

Today I'm an artist and I paint abstract and abstract figure paintings. Each piece of art I create comes with an original poem handwritten by me on the back. I use mostly acrylic and watercolor mediums. Each piece of art is inspired by my daily life, things I've been through and things I observe. I also feel that each piece is a different thought, emotion or side of me. When I am creating it's like I'm in a meditative state. I feel so calm and relaxed.

Some people might think of all that I've been through as a negative but I think of it as a positive. It's made me a better and stronger person and I wouldn't change a thing. I do admit I have good days and I also have bad days when I want to just cry. Not because I feel sorry for myself but it can be hard sometimes living in this world today where society tells you that you have to look or be a certain way. I believe we are more than just our bodies, we are the souls within. I also have days where I have the passion and inspiration to create but my body doesn't want to cooperate and requires more rest. This can be very frustrating at times. My main goal as an artist, a writer, and a person is to help and inspire others. Today, I still work with the Make A Wish Foundation by donating some of my art for their auctions and by donating part of the proceeds from my art sales to them.

95

"I am an artist and a writer creating in a world full of chaos. Overcoming a brain tumor and other obstacles and challenges through art and poetry."

Sierra Barnes

<u>Fight Of My Life</u>
<u>By Sierra Barnes</u>

Life ain't always easy
we stumble and we fall
I cry out
as I try to get around these walls

The ones that sometimes
cave in on me
but in spite of it all
I got to believe

There's a spark
in the sky
I can't explain
call me crazy
but trust me I'm okay
day by day
night by night
this journey that I'm on
this fight of my life.

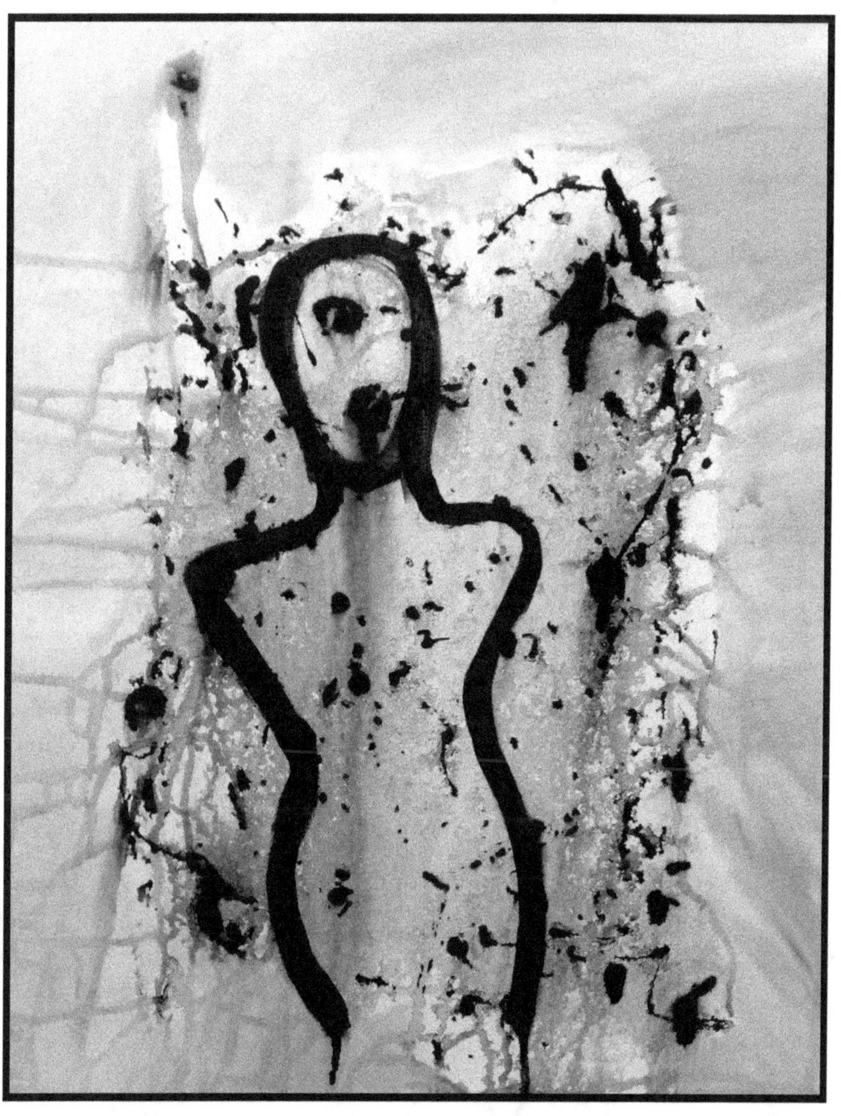

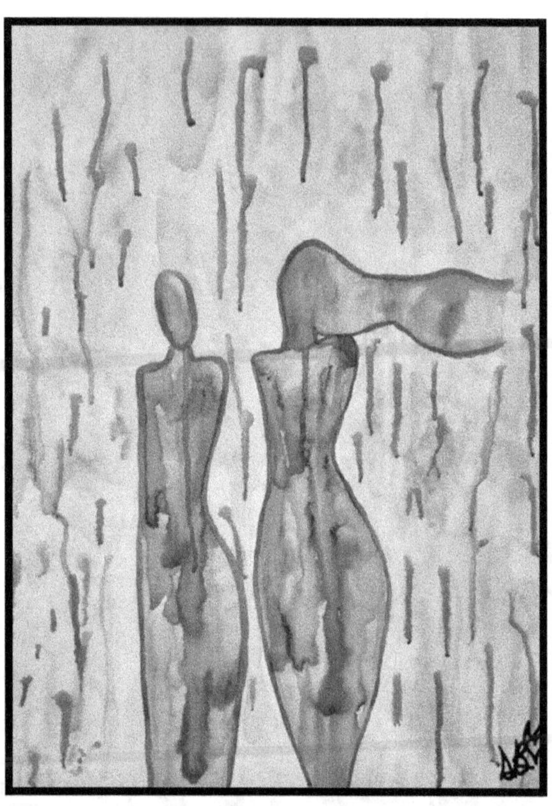

Commotion
By Sierra Barnes

Going through
our own commotion
In our bodies, minds, and souls

We somehow work through
A fight in the dark
Making our way through it
Determination and heart

Somehow it works out fine
Even when I panic
Feeling terrified
Anxiety and Self-doubt

Breaking through
my own commotion
In my body, mind, and soul.

<u>Living With Beautiful Imperfections</u>
<u>By Sierra Barnes</u>

Thrown down for imperfections
I'm a star in the wind
they say I should be going
in the other direction
trying to make it to the sky
as the storms burst
I awake only to find
my self-worth

Speak what you want
speak what you will
I'll just turn away
bringing myself forward
to live another day

We are souls
more than skin and bones
living with beautiful imperfections.

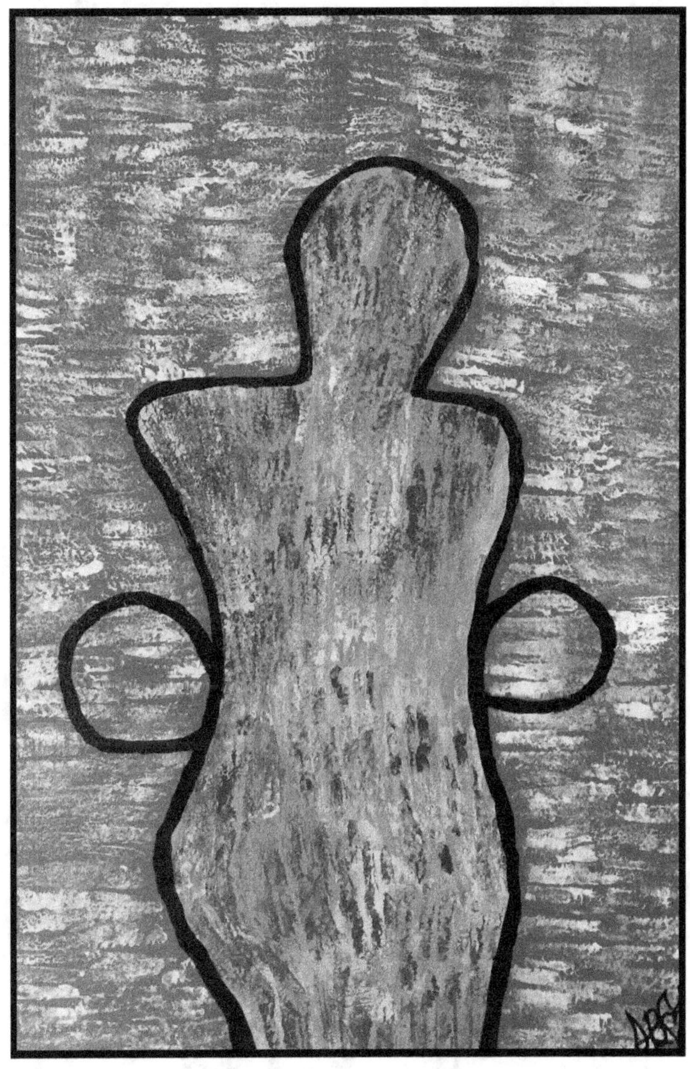

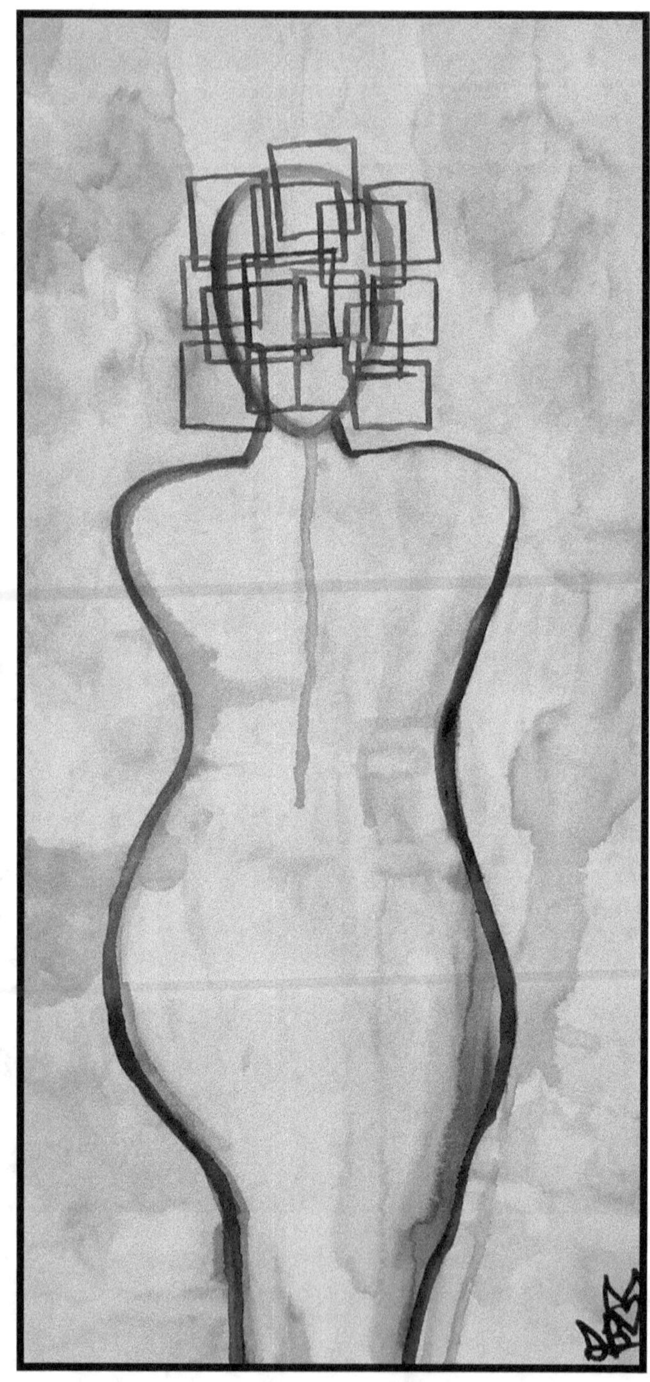

Wave
By Sierra Barnes

Some days
I'm a wreck
Stuck in my head
Still dealing with it all

I know it's an illusion
Some might say
there are simple solutions

To this mess
The one in my head
Invading my space

I know
it's meant for growth
Something greater unknown

I will ride out this wave
The wave in my head
Making me a mess.

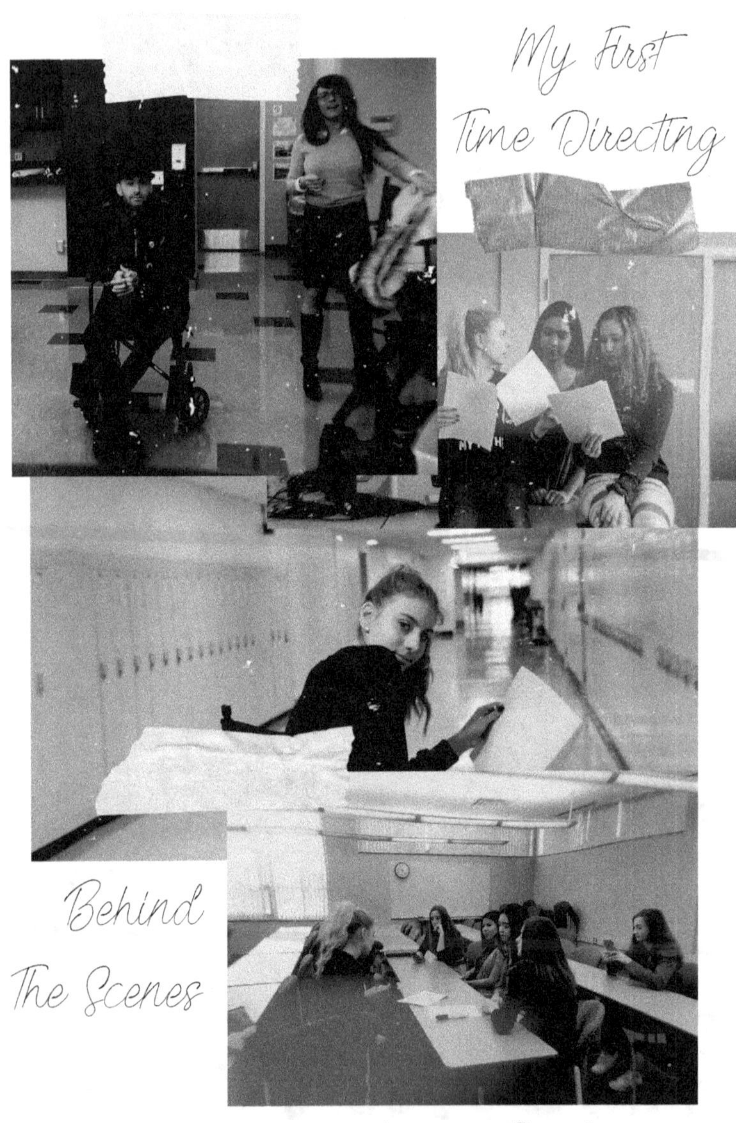
My First
Time Directing

Behind
The Scenes

"Starlight Tours"

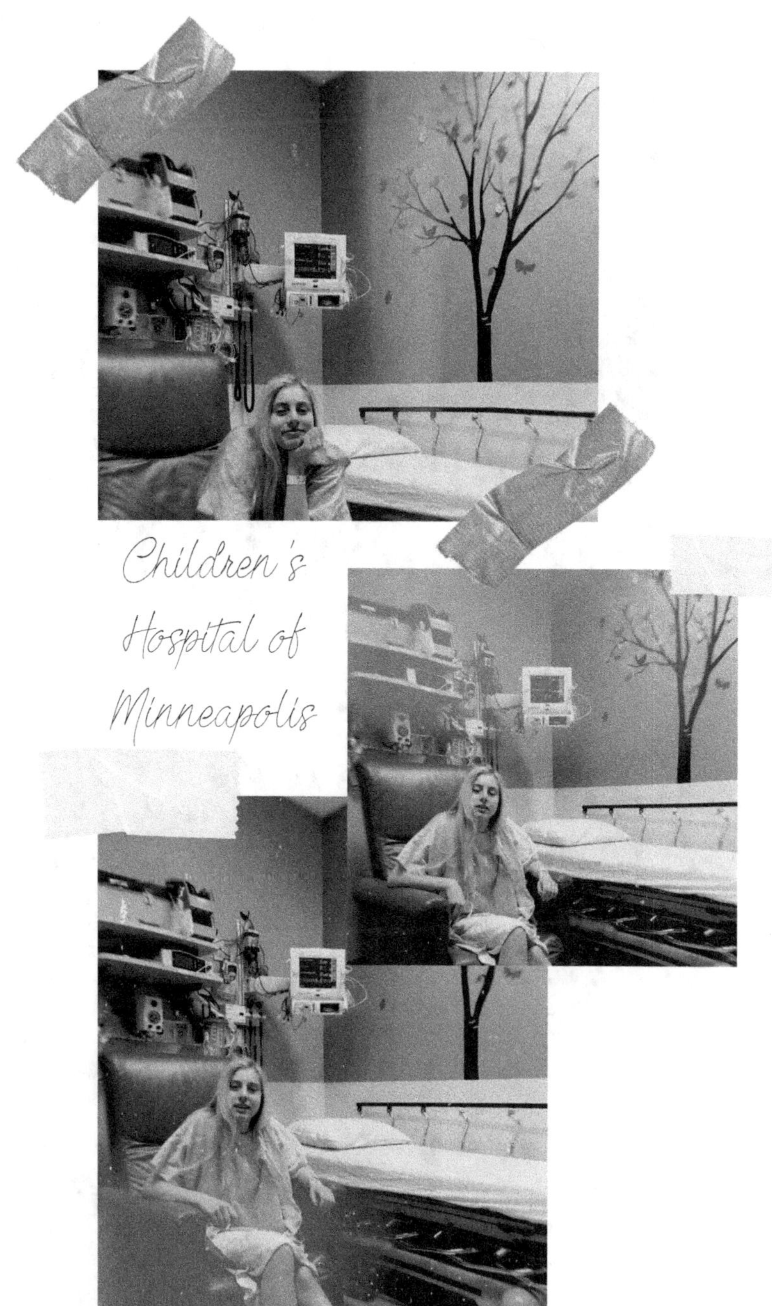
Children's
Hospital of
Minneapolis

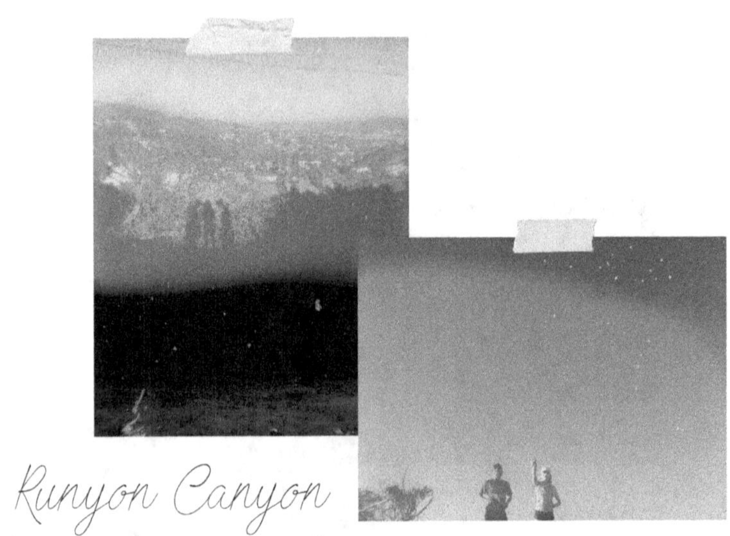

Runyon Canyon

Emily

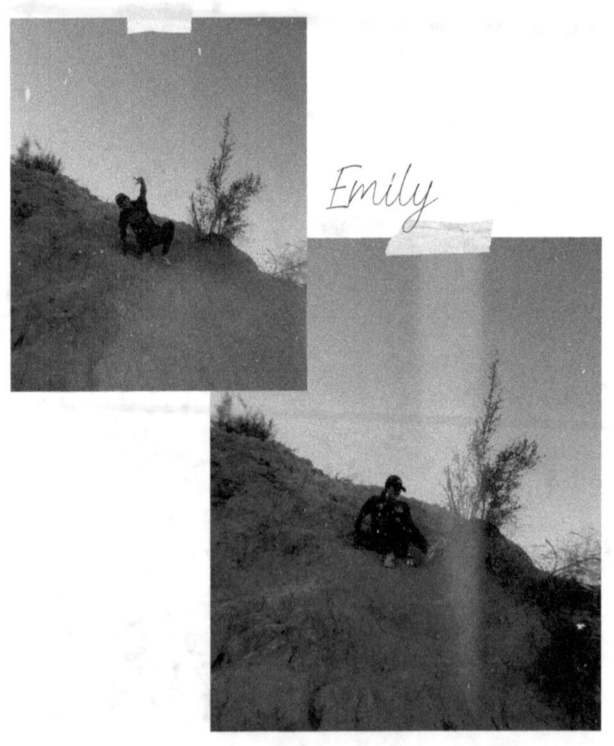

Behind
The Scenes

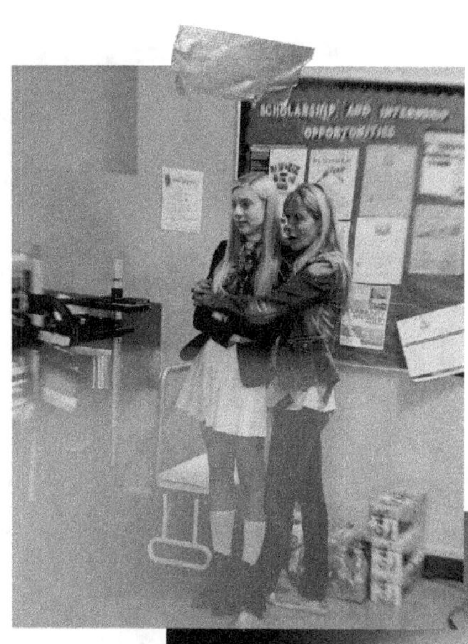

"Gradiate"

Cannes Film Festival
Cannes, France

Last spring I had the amazing opportunity to head off to Cannes, France for the Cannes Film Festival. I went to Cannes because I was nominated for two awards for the film I starred in, "Clockmaker." We ended up winning both! I won Best Young Talent and the film won Festival Director's Choice.

The rest of our trip was filled with a bunch of events, exploring, walking in fashion shows and photoshoots.

While there, I absolutely fell in love with the culture and lifestyle. I had been to Paris before, but Cannes was completely different. The whole living style was based on relaxation and health. The beach was across the street from us; the water was shockingly blue. There were fruits and vegetables galore; it was almost impossible to find junk food. Plus, the daily flea markets were a bonus.

Cannes was truly a life changing experience and I cant wait to go back next year!

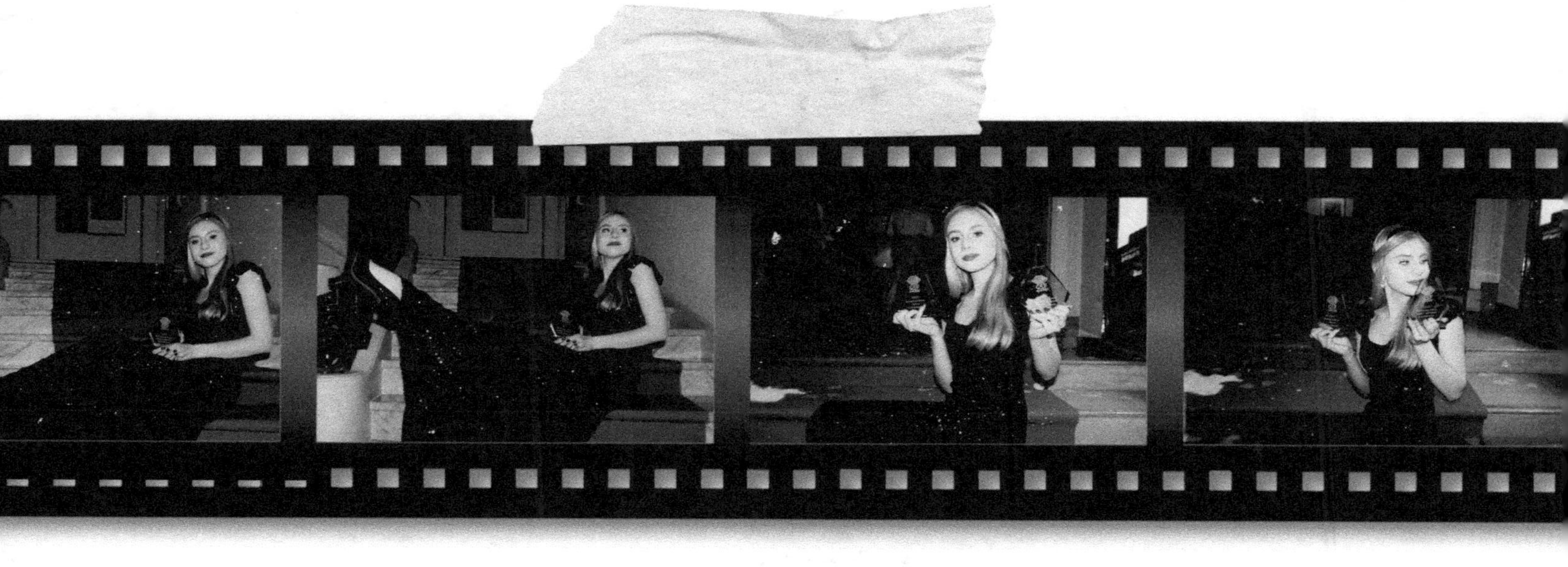

Cannes, France

Met Gala

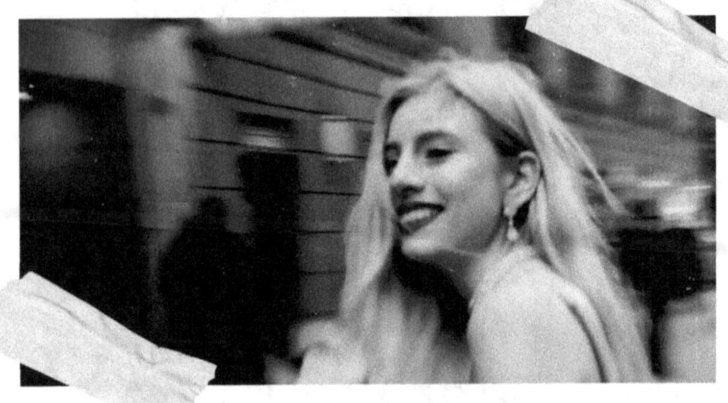

New York City

Zendaya

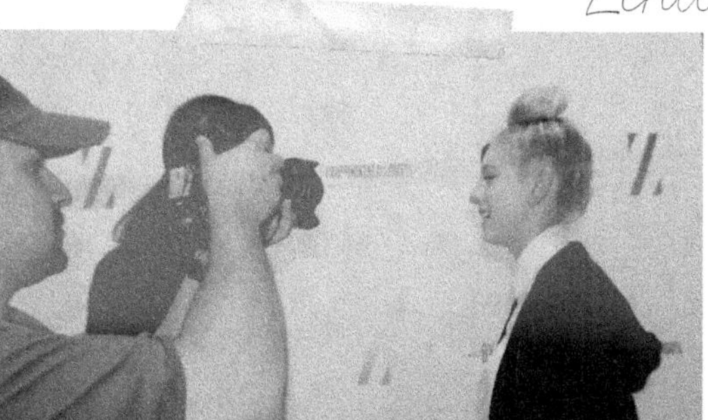

DxZ Clothing Launch

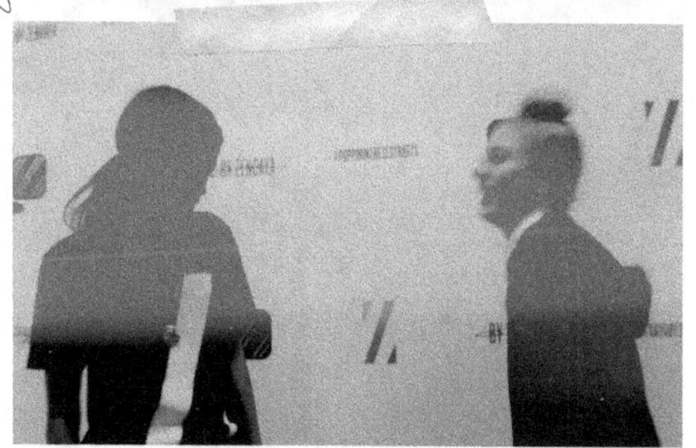

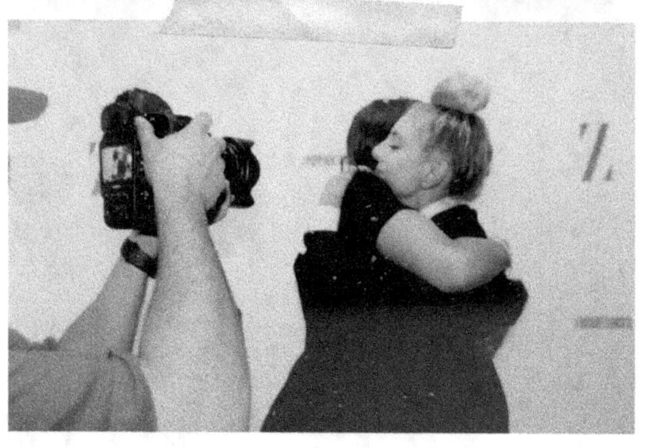

Madison Williams

Grade III Anaplastic Ependymoma Survivor

Madison

My name is Madison and I live in Georgia. I was an ordinary 16 year old girl; I loved to hang out with my friends, go to movies, ride horses and run. I loved playing piano, guitar, mandolin, and clarinet. I loved singing and writing my own songs. I wanted to grow up to be an orthopedic surgeon. My life changed drastically in March of 2016, my sophomore year in high school. I had a massive headache for three weeks but I didn't think much of it because teenage girls have many, many reasons to have headaches. It could have been my menstrual cycle or hormones or even a cold.

At the end of those three weeks, my mom and I were walking into Target to pick up some things for our girls night -- when the guys aren't home, my mom and I eat brownies and fruit for dinner and watch movies. As we walked through the dollar aisle, I stopped and had to hold on to the wall to stay upright. When my mom asked me what was wrong, I replied saying that it felt like an ice pick had hit me in my left eye. I quickly got it back together and finished shopping with my mom and we went home and had our girls night and watched our movie. But my headache never left.

The next morning, **March 19, 2016**, my headache woke me up and I couldn't stop crying. My dad ran in and I started throwing up. He went and got my mom who is a doctor of physical therapy. She came in and helped me to the living room couch and gave me a trashcan in case I kept throwing up. My parents started going back and forth about "maybe it's the flu" or "maybe a virus". There was a stomach virus going around and a lot of my mom's patients had to cancel their appointments that week. My mom, however, had a fear that she kept to herself. She told my dad that she was going to take me to the quick care nearby but started to explain in the car that she was taking me instead to the emergency room because she was afraid there was something wrong with my brain and she wanted a CT scan of my head.

On the ride there I started playing with my right hand and my mom looked over and asked "What are you doing?"

"That's so weird..."
"What's weird?"
"My hand is numb and tingling."
"Are you ok?"
"Hehe, yeah. Now my right leg is numb..." I began slurring, "and the right side of my face!" She began to speed as her worries about me having a brain tumor were playing out in front of her.

When we arrived at the emergency room, the whole right side of my body head to toe was numb and I couldn't walk. She had to drag me in and sit me in a chair where I shook and threw up in my trash can. They immediately put me in a wheelchair and took me back while my mom was still checking in. They took me to the CT scan machine and took a scan of my head.

After rolling me back to my room the technician told us that it would probably be about twenty minutes before the doctor was in with the results. Five minutes later the doctor came in, sat down, and sighed at the floor. I can still remember the look on my mom's face and she later told me that it felt like she had ice water dumped on her. He looked at us and said that I had a brain tumor and massive swelling on the left side of my brain. He asked if she wanted to see the images because he knew about her medical education. The images showed a calcified tumor about the size of a golf ball located in the left parietal lobe just posterior to the motor strip with the entire left side of my brain swollen.

My mom called my dad who was at a soccer game by then and she was ok until he answered the phone. I had been unbothered by the tumor because I wasn't thinking about the future, I was thinking, "ok, what do I have to do next." Because of that, I took the phone from her and said, "Hey Daddy, I have a brain tumor." My mom freaked out and took the phone from me and began explaining. He was forty-five minutes away but somehow made it to the emergency room within twenty-five minutes. He had just enough time to hold my hand before they rolled me out to the helicopter that took me to Children's Healthcare of Atlanta at Scottish Rite.

I always smiled because I felt like it would comfort others to think I wasn't so scared or in so much pain. What's the use in scaring people who can't take it away? I stayed there for three days while they gave me many medicines through an IV to try to decrease the amount of swelling in my brain. There was so much swelling that they couldn't operate.

Then, on March 22, I had a six hour brain surgery to remove the tumor. They were able to do a complete resection of the tumor and I recovered from surgery so well that I was discharged about a week later! They told us that they are very sure that it was a cancer called Ependymoma. Although I was recovering "very well" I still felt horrible. I couldn't read even a greeting card or focus on coloring or my head would start to hurt very badly. Visitors made me exhausted no matter how much or how little I interacted with them. The mix of narcotic painkillers, anti-seizure and other medicines on top of having my head cut into was not pleasant in the slightest.

I had to sit in the front seat of the car on our way back home almost lying flat with the darkest sunglasses on because light, noises and the slightest bumps in the road were so painful. I cried most of that ride, and slept from exhaustion the other parts. My mom called ahead to my favorite Italian restaurant and we stopped and picked up one of my favorite meals on our way home and I laid on the couch. We ate with my Granddaddy and my older brother in the living room so that I could stay on the couch.

I laid there on that couch for two weeks visiting with people, sleeping and eating. My mom would bathe me, help me around the house when I couldn't use the walker (also with her help), and sit, giving me my medicines and antibacterial creams. I had so many that we kept a basket next to me on the coffee table with all of my medicines in it.

My mom started doing what we always do (but always shouldn't!) by researching Ependymoma. Though my neurosurgeon told my mom that he was pretty sure that's what it was, he made her promise not to research it because he wanted us to wait until the biopsy returned and we had a definitive diagnosis. But, really -- who is going to wait??

There are three grades of Ependymomas.

Grade I tumors are either Subependymomas or Myxopapillary Ependymomas. Both are typically slow growing tumors and both are benign.

Grade II Ependymomas are also benign but do require a small amount of treatment after surgery to ensure that everything is gone.

Then there is Grade III, Anaplastic Ependymoma. This is the malignant form.

Ependymoma is a rare type of cancer with only 250 pediatric cases a year, and for my age group, only 50 a year. Fifty a year! Because of Ependymoma's rarity, there is no known cause or a known treatment plan. There are, however, treatments that are fairly effective. This is what we found when we researched while waiting to hear for sure what type of cancer my tumor was. We received a call from one neuro-oncologists, Dr. A, and she started off by telling us what grade of Ependymoma I was diagnosed with. She informed us that I had Grade III Anaplastic Ependymoma, the malignant form. She let us know that this meant that it could have also spread to my spine because it affects the ependymal cells - which line the brain, are in the center of the brain, and are in our spines. She wanted to do something called a spinal tap which lets them test my spinal fluid to see if there were any cancerous cells present there. She also said that these cancer cells do not react to chemotherapy so we had to do something more aggressive: radiation. She suggested that we do proton beam radiation because it is more precise with its beams, thus being more safe to the surrounding parts of the brain because they would receive less of the beams that stray away. The only problem with that was that they didn't have proton radiation in Georgia yet.

My parents told her that if they had to fly us to Australia to receive treatment they would. They wanted the best care. She told them that there are three places that we could choose from: Boston, Jacksonville, or Houston. She told them that we needed to pick which we wanted her to send my case to and hope that they had an opening because she felt it was mandatory that I start radiation in less than 30 days.

She said that the one in Boston was the newest one and had a good track record, the one in Houston was older but also had a good track record, and that a lot of Georgians choose to go to Jacksonville because it was closer. Because of the fact that the one in Houston had been practicing for longer and had a good track record, that is the one we chose. Dr. A. said that she had a friend who worked at the one in Houston and she would get on the phone immediately to see if she could get me in. We got on a plane on Friday, went around Houston looking for an apartment to move to for my radiation treatments, then flew back home to say our farewells.

My treatment started that next Monday and lasted for seven weeks. The facility was MD Anderson. We went to the radiation center and they marked on my face and had me lay down as they put a heated plastic mask over my head and it molded itself to the exact shape of my face. I had a mouthpiece in while they did it and it always made me think of a lime green Darth Vader mask. They would play The Beatles radio in the gantry because they are my favorite band and would do everything they could to make sure I was ok and comfortable. That metal table however couldn't be made comfortable because they needed to know exactly that the beam was hitting the exact part of my brain that it was supposed to.

In the main hospital building they would take my blood once a week to do their labs. I would talk to another doctor about how I was doing and they would give me medicines for my nausea, or pain, or dizziness. I currently have the whole neuro test memorized. 'Squeeze my fingers, walk on your heels, now walk on your toes, tandem walking, follow my finger with your eyes...'

We tried to do fun things while we were there like going out to eat, going to the zoo and going to the mall. But for the most part, I was too fatigued or in too much pain to walk everywhere so they wheeled me around in a wheelchair. The two things that I loved and that I now miss so badly are eating in Rice Village with my mom and going on an afternoon trip to Galveston with my best friend, Emily. She flew out to us after she had finished school that spring. She and I have been inseparable from before kindergarten so it was natural that she would be with me. Those last two weeks were better because she was there. She helped me get my mind off of it and also was my cheerleader when I needed her support.

On the last day of treatment I got to sign the wall in the proton center and ring the gong. It felt good but wasn't that relieving feeling that I had hoped it would be because cancer still looms over me now. With my type of brain cancer, we don't know if I'm cured or not. If not, it could come back next month or when I'm fifty. There is never an "all clear" or a day when I get to hold the sign saying "Cancer Free." I have a thirty percent chance of a recurrence at any point in my lifetime.

We drove all the way back to Georgia in June of 2017, where I got to see my granddad and brother again. I had a bunch of friends come over and hangout. Daily activities were distracting and, overall, things were looking up.

I started to see things in my room at night when we were in Houston but I could blink and they would be gone. I never told anyone until January of 2017, when I couldn't make them go away. They were terrifying. I would mostly see the silhouette of a tall man with a hat walking towards me, but also saw silhouettes of little girls, or even silhouettes of non human creatures that would be best described as Gollum from Lord Of The Rings. I always felt like they wanted to hurt or kill me. My parents found out by me screaming in the middle of the night and crying because I was so scared. They had me sleep in their room with them for a while on the couch. Then weeks turned into months and I ended up spending all of my nights for 2017 in their room (don't worry -- they moved a bed into their room so I didn't sleep on a couch for a year!). I would see things run at me from the bathroom and the worst one that still makes me cry when I think about it was when I was closing the shutters on one of the windows and saw a grotesquely mutilated face staring back at me. It made me fall backwards onto the floor and panic for about an hour. I still won't look at the windows when I shut them at night. I began to have separation anxiety and would sit in the back of my mom's clinic and stay there during the day because I couldn't be home alone out of fear of another hallucination. I even began hearing things. One day I was walking up the stairs in an empty house to grab my golf clothes before practice. My granddad was in the car in the garage. As I reached the middle of the staircase, I heard my dad's voice yell at me not to go upstairs. I collapsed on the stairs and began to cry out of fear because I knew he was in Florida on a business trip.

They took me to a psychologist who ended up telling me that I needed an emotional support dog (and we got one!), but I ended up feeling uncomfortable with her because I felt like she judged me. We quit going to her and then later found a psychiatrist whom I love and still go to. The dog, however, I still have and love him dearly. He is the reason I am comfortable being home alone during the day time. His name is Toby and he is an amazing dog. I intend on having him Emotional Support Animal and Therapy Dog certified after much training so that I can take him to hospitals for kids to cuddle and pet.

Currently I still struggle with PTSD, anxiety, claustrophobia and my health because of Anaplastic Ependymoma. It is very easy for me to get sick due to my compromised immune system which is scary during flu season because the flu could be dangerous for me. I also struggle with my regular MRIs, which will be lifelong, because of the PTSD and claustrophobia. I can't get in an MRI tube or even a CT scan because they trigger panic attacks for me. I have to be sedated which scares my father.

Even though I am still in pain because of what happened over two years ago, I am still pushing. I am inspired by all the other survivors because I can understand a little better what they are going through. I want to help them which is why I changed what I want to be from an orthopedic surgeon to a neurosurgeon.

I learned about the Pediatric Brain Tumor Foundation and the first event we did with them was the Starry Night 5K - I had a blast! It was amazing and touching for me to be able to see and meet many other kids who like me who have had tumors. I knew that I wanted to help them. I then participated in the Couture for Kids fashion show. I was very nervous to start with, but had a blast and met awesome people like Grace and a little four year old girl who always inspires me. She is one of my favorite people on this planet. She and I had an instant connection and still see each other. It wasn't until we were doing a video together for fundraising for the PBTF that I learned that her brain tumor was also Grade III Anaplastic Ependymoma.

I also help out at the Christmas Party for brain tumor survivors held by the PBTF every year and even performed at the next Starry Night 5K. I performed an original song that I wrote about my experience with my cancer. I named it Superman because everyone I knew was posting the Superman logo with an 'M' instead of an 'S' in support of me when I had my brain surgery. I'm so thankful for the Pediatric Brain Tumor Foundation and what they do. They have made a world of difference for me and for my family.

I'm also thankful to say, I'm a survivor.

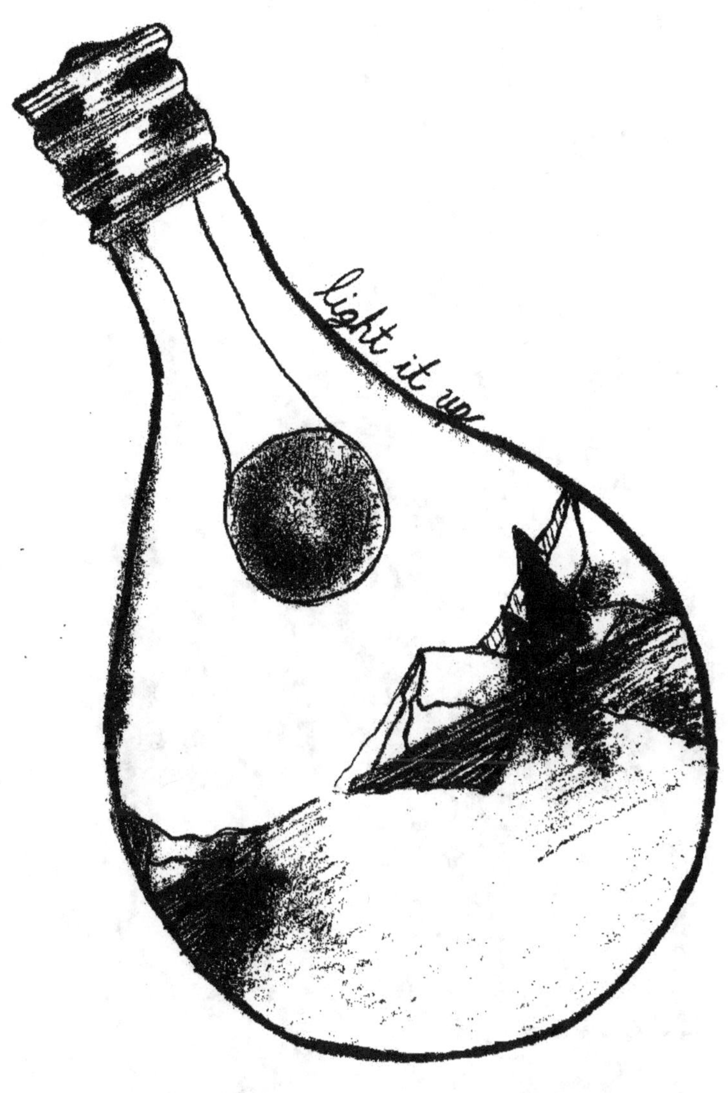

Sketch By Grace Wethor

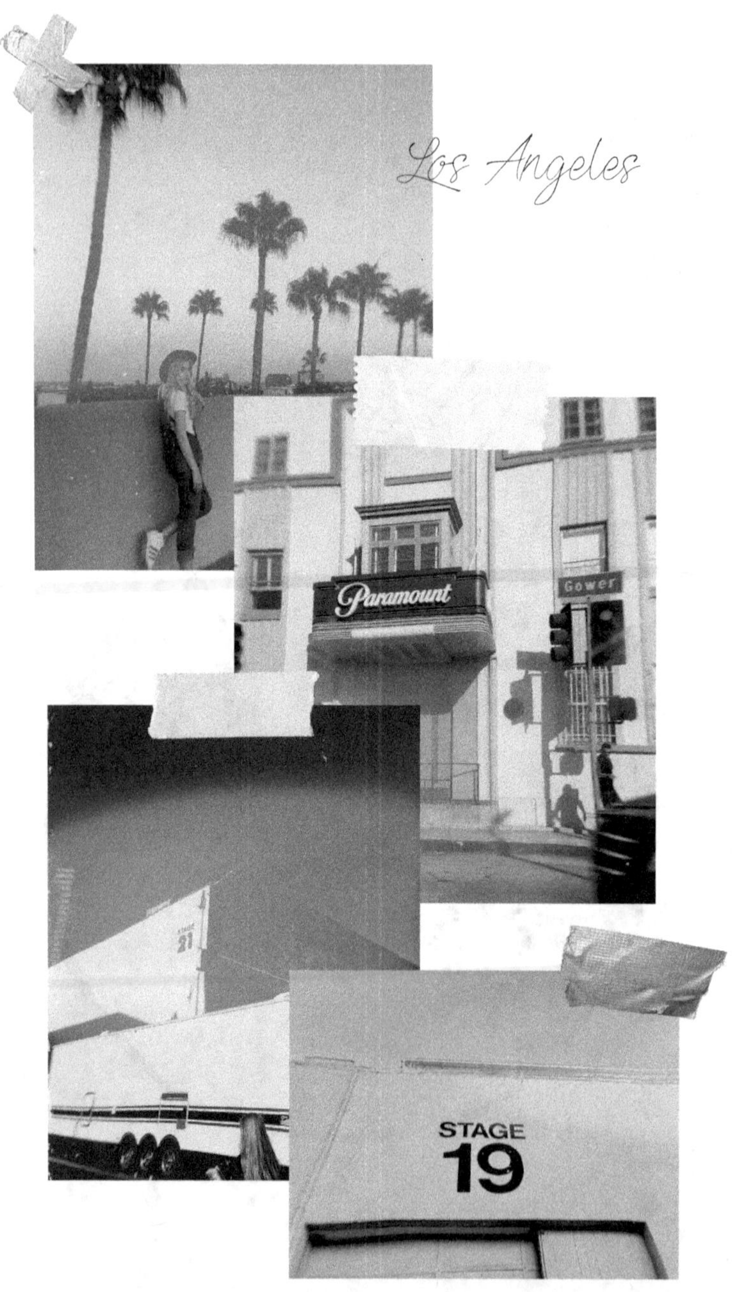
Los Angeles
Paramount
Gower
STAGE
19

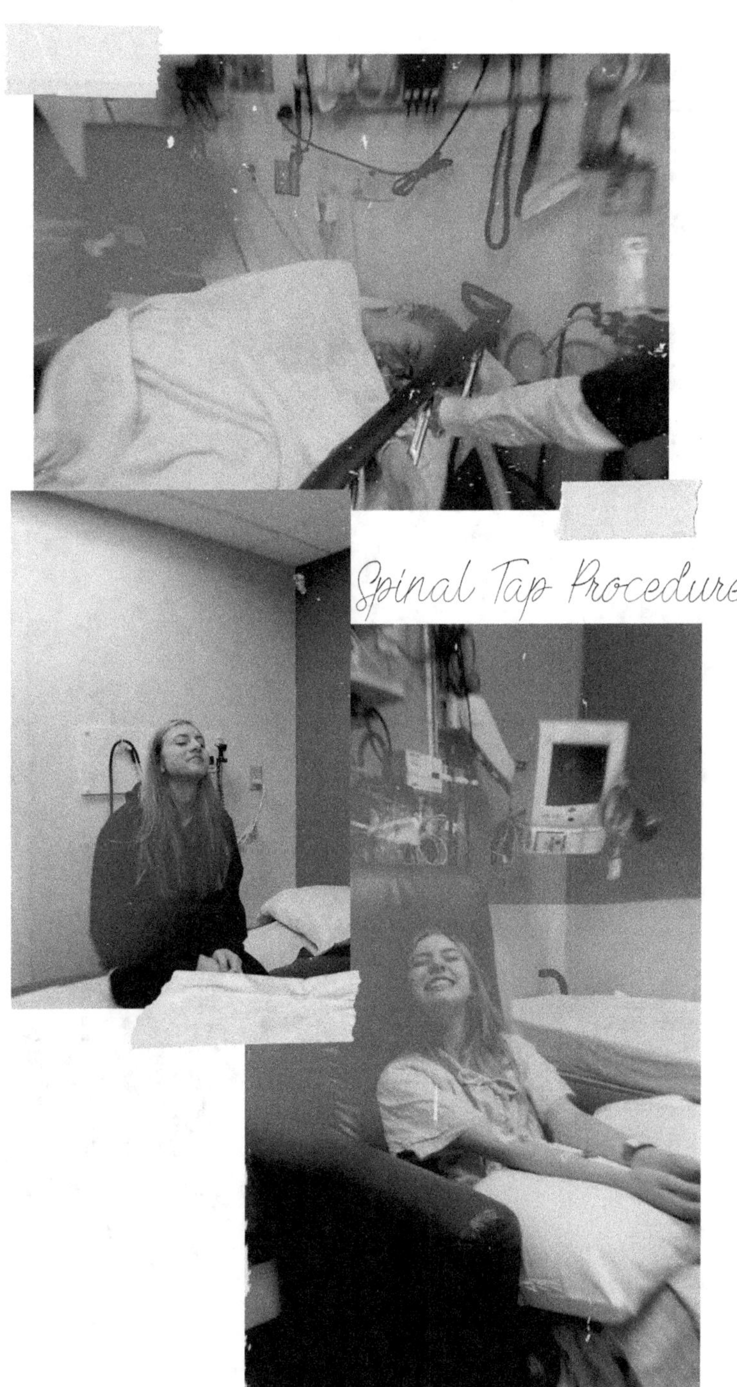
Spinal Tap Procedure

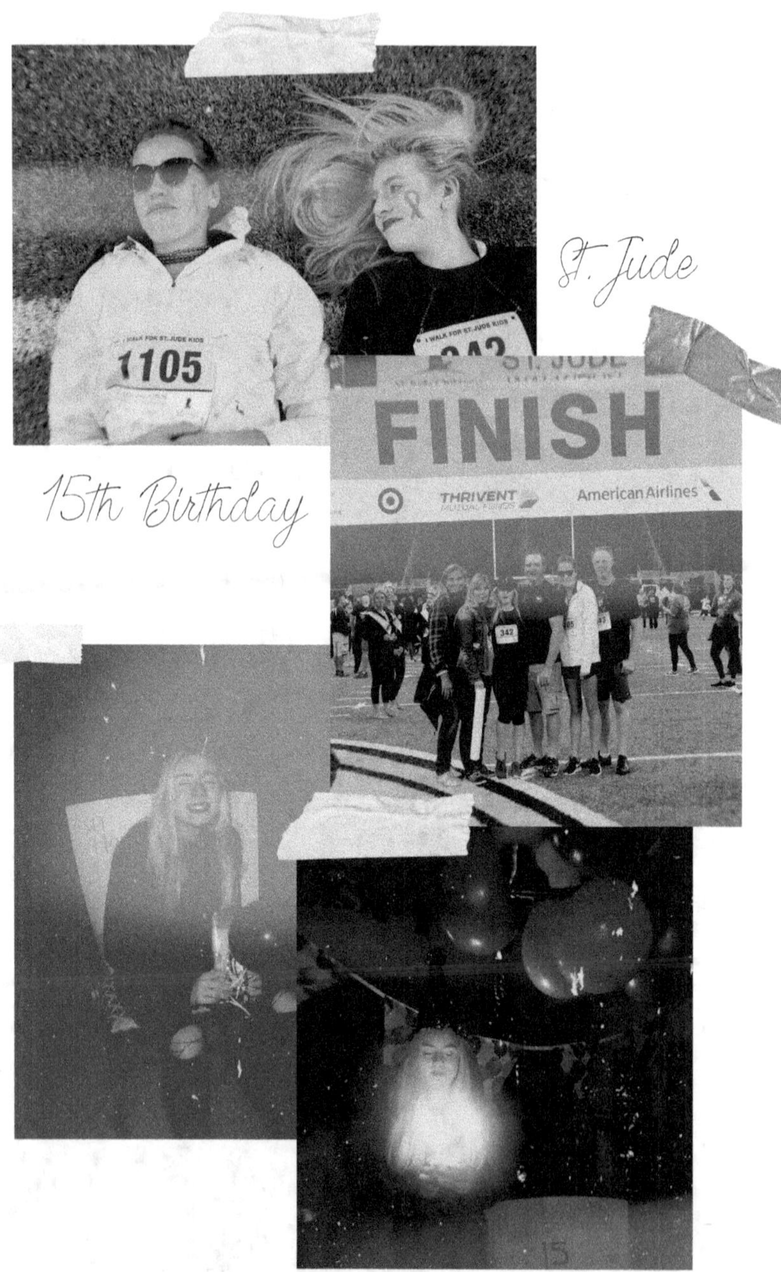
15th Birthday
St. Jude
1105
FINISH
THRIVENT
MUTUAL FUNDS
American Airlines
342

15th Birthday With St. Jude
US Bank Stadium - Downtown Minneapolis, MN

For my 15th birthday, I had the amazing opportunity to team up with St. Jude for The Walk To End Childhood Cancer on September 24th, 2016. It was in my hometown of Minneapolis, so I caught the red eye from LA and landed at 3 am. If you look at the two photos on the bottom, you can see me delusionally smiling as my mom forces me to blow out candles at 3:30 in the morning. I took a quick nap and then headed downtown for our 7 am start. The event was HUGE and so many people came to support. It was amazing to see the whole community coming together to make a difference.

Truly a birthday I will never forget.

Pediatric Brain Tumor Foundation Fashion Show

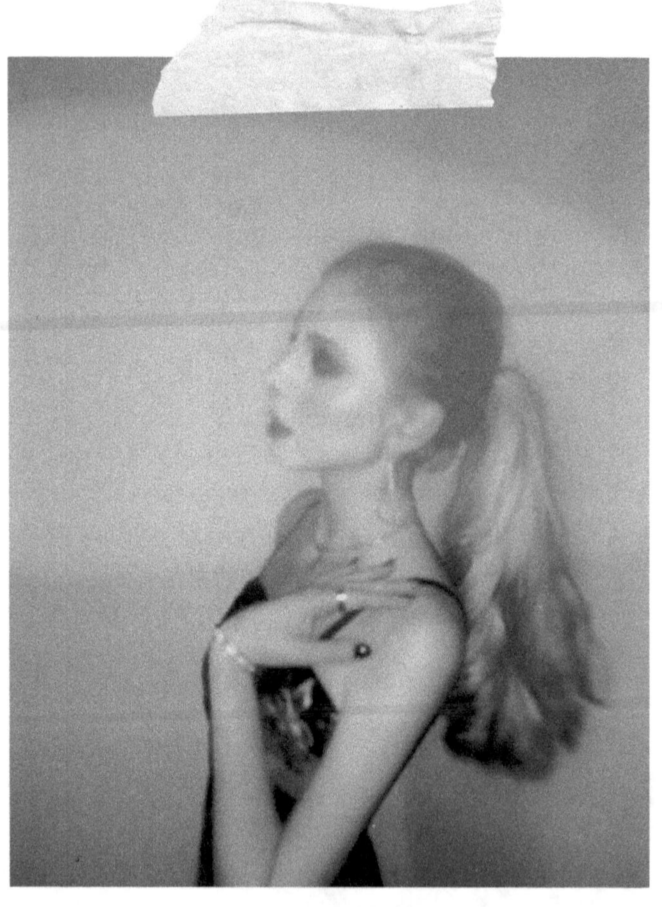

Atlanta, GA

Black Hearts Ball

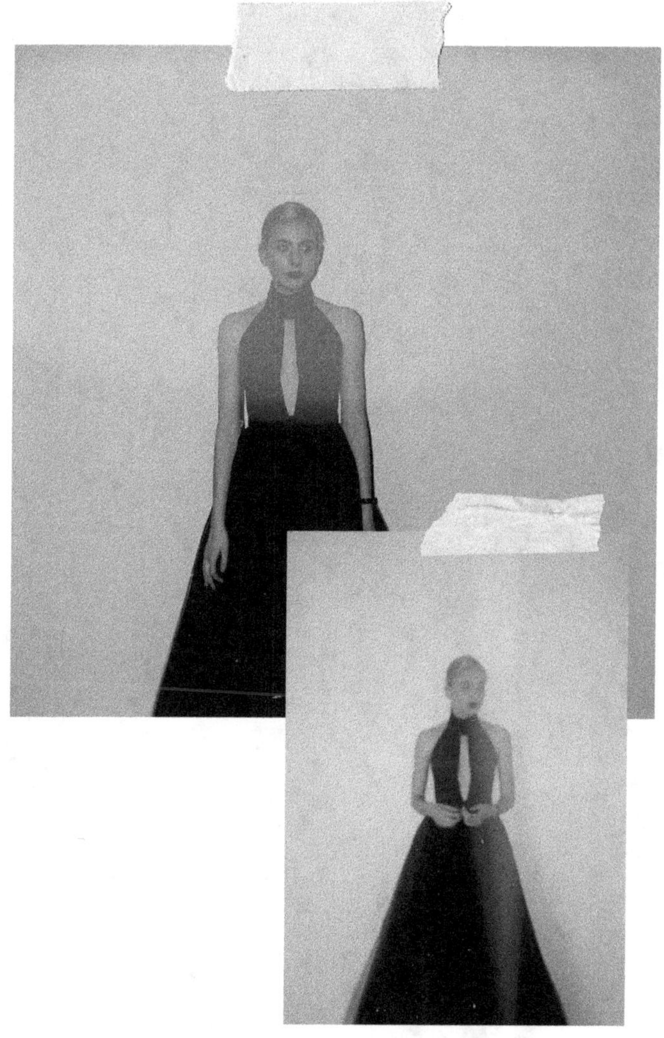

Minneapolis, MN

133

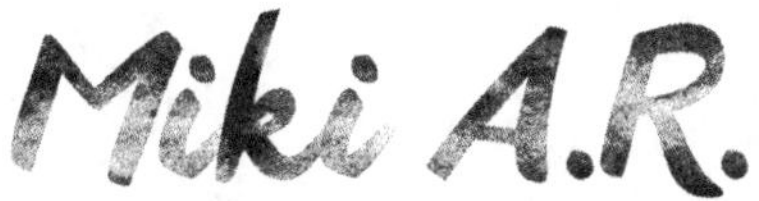

Neurofibromatosis Survivor

Miki

My story isn't the the expected type of situation when it comes to finding out about a brain tumor or being a survivor. I didn't start feeling ill or have a seizure. I didn't have a scan for another reason, I didn't have questionable blood tests or any other medical testing. I didn't have any of those scenarios because I was born with my condition, which is Neurofibromatosis. Neurofibromatosis is also known as "NF". It is a genetic disorder that affects one in approximately every 2,800 people. There are three types of NF: NF1, NF2, and Schwannomatosis. I have NF1.

Research shows that those with NF1 occasionally might have tumors develop in the brain, on cranial nerves or on the spinal cord. While they stress the word "occasionally", these areas happen to be exactly where all of my tumors are, in addition to many other areas. That must make me the one "Occasional" NF patient with the exact genetic make-up to have not just one, but all of those tumors. NF tumors are generally not cancerous. They can cause health problems by pressing on nearby areas, which then cause secondary issues. Sometimes a benign (non-cancer) tumor may become malignant (cancerous), but most people with NF1 will never develop a malignant tumor. Still, they can cause significant neurological symptoms depending on their size and location near other structures in the brain and spine. Some benign tumors can progress to become malignant. So far, although my brain tumors are actively growing, they are slow growing and benign. I have honestly been blessed!

My story begins when I was 7 weeks old. My mom noticed several brown spots on me in various places that looked similar to bruises. They were not there when I was born. When my mom asked my pediatrician about the spots (what we call ladybug kisses), my doctor wrote down "Neurofibromatosis" on a post-it note and asked my mom to look it up. Then, if my mom thought the symptoms were similar to mine, to let her know.

When reading, my mom was devastated as most new parents would be. She called my doctor and she set up an appointment with a Geneticist at Texas Children's Hospital. At 9 months, the doctors visually confirmed their belief that I did in fact have NF. They then ran a blood test to check my genes. The test came back four months later as positive. It was determined that I had a more severe form of NF, even though I was the first in my family to have it. Yes, that's right. No one else in my family has NF of any form. I have what's called "Spontaneous NF 1". Meaning I'm the first in my family to have it. So on top of being an "occasional NF'er with the occasional tumors" as earlier mentioned, I am also the first in all of our family. The doctors thought that was almost impossible, so they ran the same blood test on my mom and dad…. Yep, I'm the only one!

Many people feel pity for me, but those people are the people who don't really know me. They don't really know that I've got this. They don't really know that

I am a fighter and have amazing strength. I have known about my genetic disorder since I was 7. Of course I knew before then of something being different, because I had countless doctors appointments but I didn't realize when I was younger that all of those trips to the doctor were out of the norm. I thought everyone went to the doctor a lot. Then when I was 5, my little brother Landon was born. I noticed I was given a lot more attention, attention he didn't get from my mom or my dad. The "attention" was me taking trips to my special hospital and seeing doctors. My brothers didn't get to do that. Then when I moved on from private daycare to elementary school, I noticed my friends didn't have to see doctors as much as me either. So I asked my mom why they don't see doctors like I do. She told me that it's because I have "bubbles" in my head. What my mom really meant was that I had tumors in my head. I realized that when I was about 9. If I asked, my mom would tell me what the doctors were saying in terms I could understand.

By the time I was 11, I had been diagnosed with Epilepsy. Most of my seizure episodes were at night, which meant my mom had to sleep with me every night. I think it may have been more upsetting for my mom because she was afraid to go to sleep at night.

In addition to epilepsy, from the time I was 4, doctors have been watching lesions and tumors and countless bright spots on my MRIs of my brain, neck, spine, etc. I've also developed migraines, hypothyroidism, and hypertension from NF. Until recently, I've had to limit my activities. There have been many days where I've slept 18 hours or had migraines. Up until the last year, I had severe nausea, dizziness, fatigue, moodiness, weak legs, seeing spots, seeing shadows, low body temp, etc. I have been on medications multiple times a day for 5 years. My life… our life, has definitely changed. I missed 2 months of school because I was not able to stay awake and was too weak to manage a full day of school. As you can imagine, I lost a lot of "friends" at school. People talked about me and said things that weren't true. It hurt a great deal and has made me more reserved when it come to who I share information with. I've also changed a lot as a person.

Thankfully, out of a lack for answers, my awesome doctors came to an agreement to find a solution. I started Botox injections over a year ago and can now manage most days. I still get 31 Botox injections every 12 weeks, and have 2-3 MRI's and attend approximately 20 doctors appointments a year. I have to take medications daily, but I am able to do what I want now!

It's not the greatest feeling being different from most others, but I knew, and still know, that my mom will always be there to support me. She takes me to every appointment. Even when we have to stay at the hospital for a week. I now have many friends, I have great grades in school and I'm even on my high school fishing team! With all that I've been through, I have been blessed with being supported by amazing people in my life. There have been so many great people that I've met. True warriors and survivors. Some you would never expect them to be, or ever of been struggling. People that I would have never met if I wasn't having a similar experience myself. Because of those people and the members of my family, I am now looking forward to a career in the medical field. I will continue, even with my current and future struggles, to look for a way to help others.

We should all be thankful for what we have, know that there is always someone out there struggling more than we are, and not be afraid to be there for others. Kindness and compassion matters. People may not know how to ask for help, but all of us will need it at some point. Be a friend.

Every day is a new day. When we wake-up, we get to make a choice to have a good day or a bad day. Make today matter.

Surviving.

M. A. R.

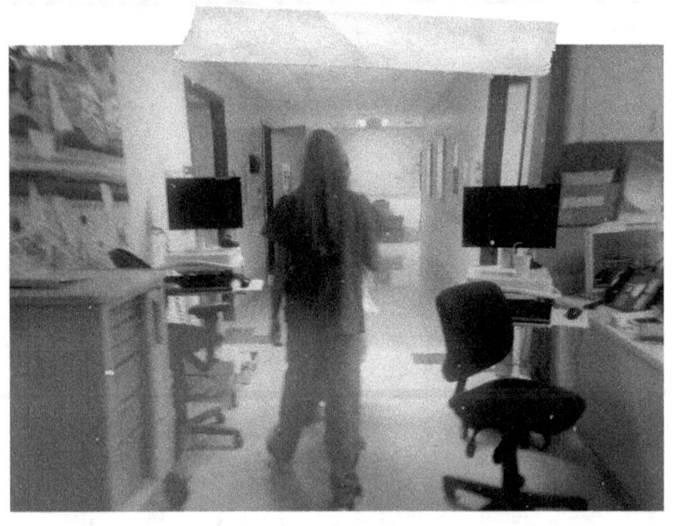

Mayo Clinic

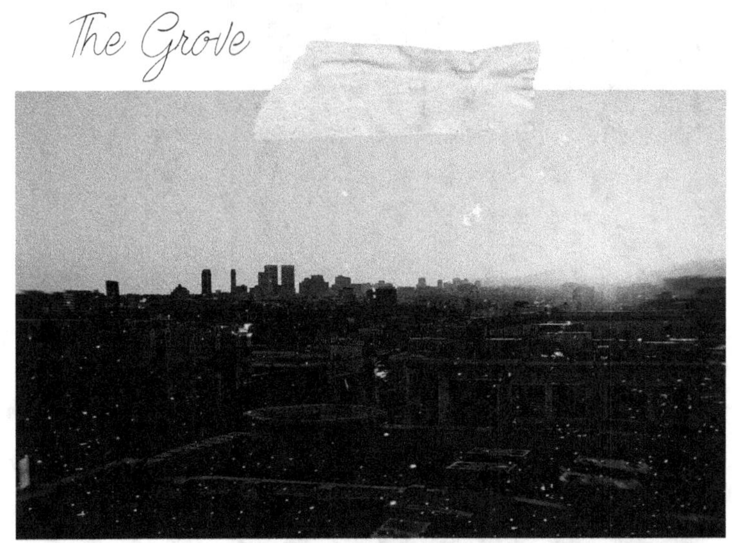

The Grove
Los Angeles

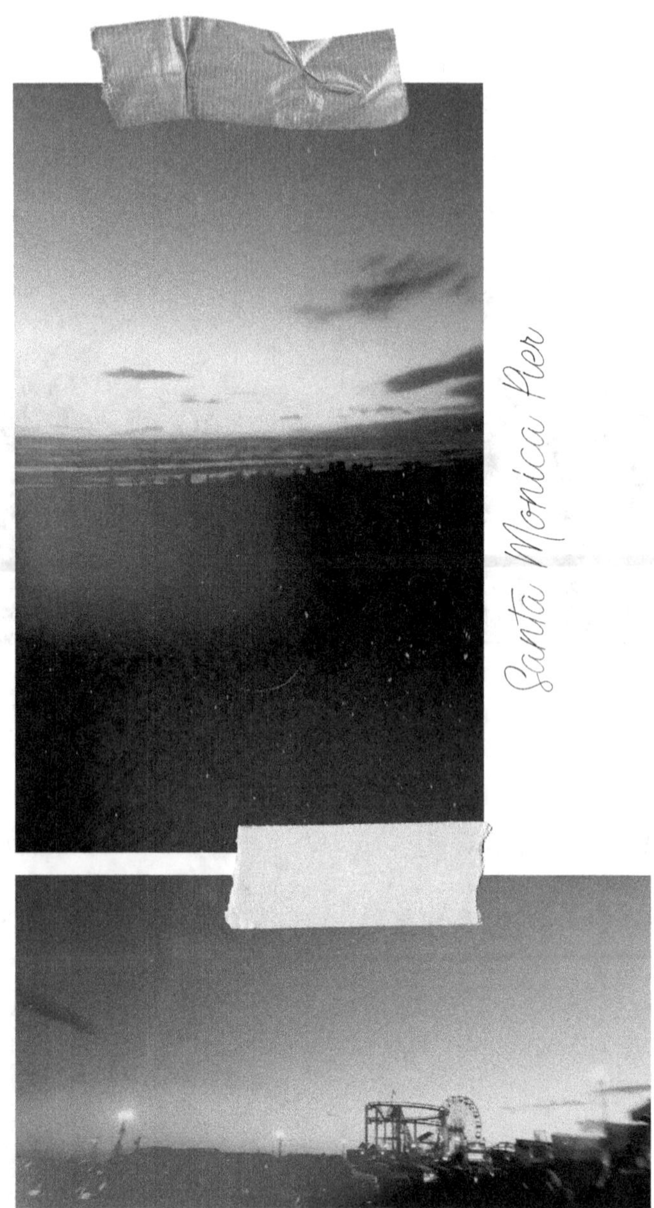
Santa Monica Pier

Downtown Los Angeles

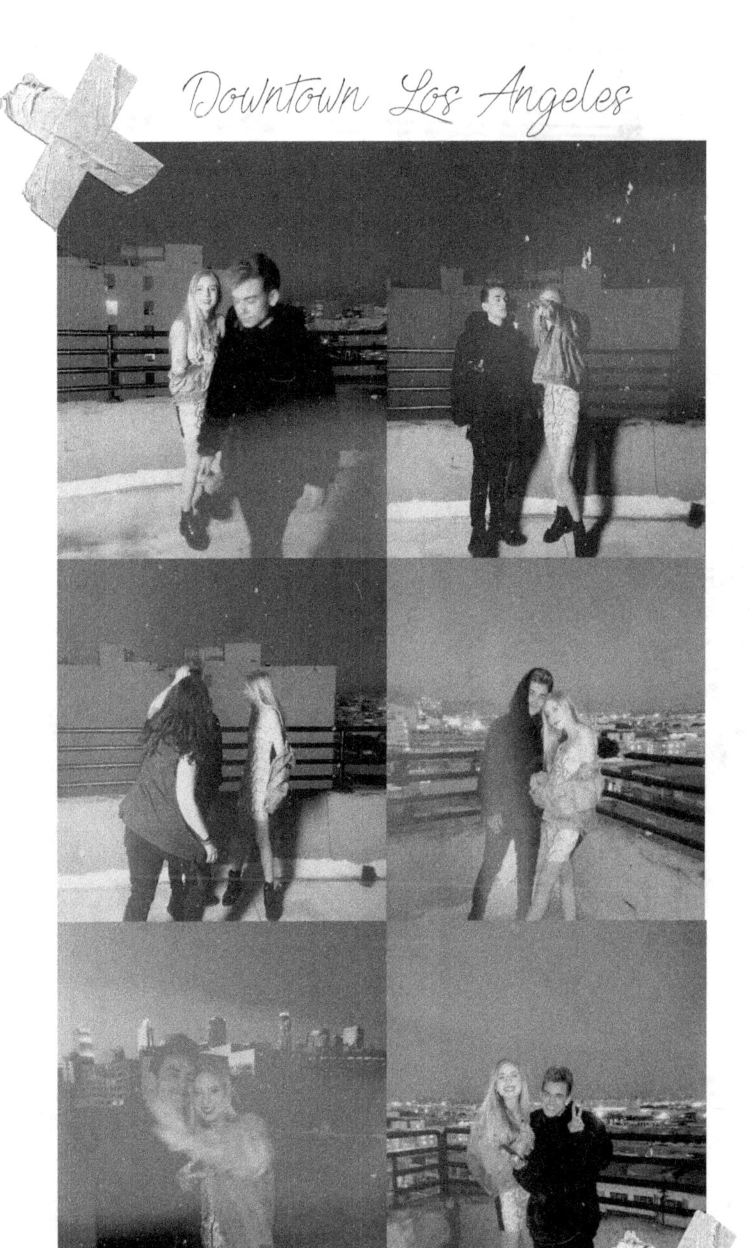

#Monument Music Video

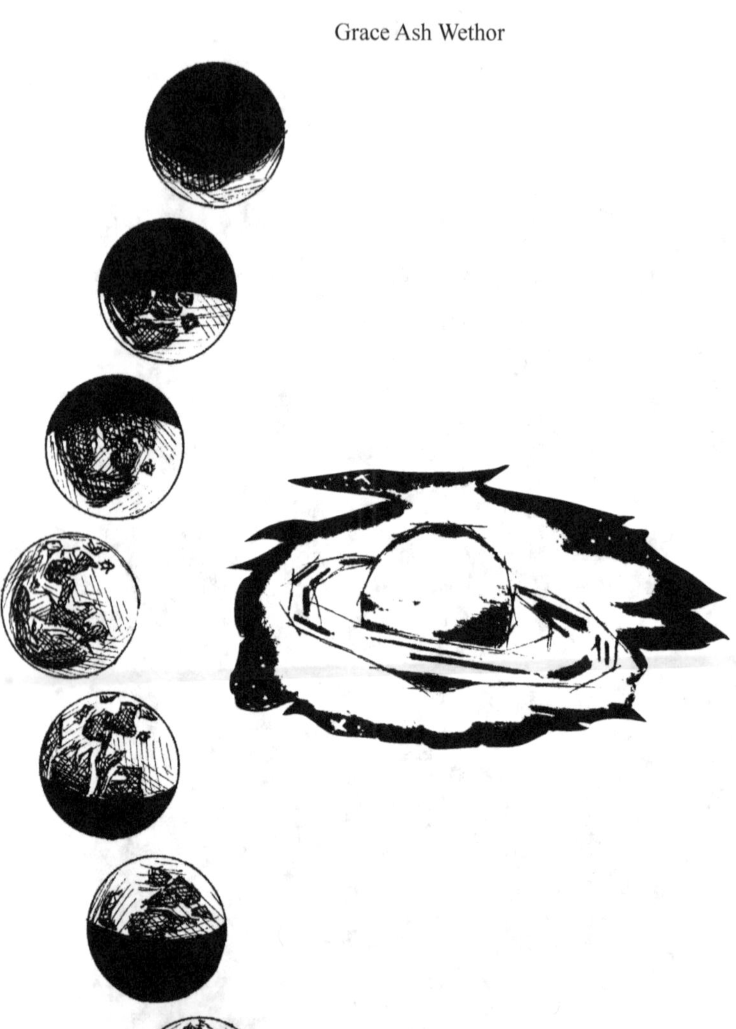

Sketch By Heather Rosati

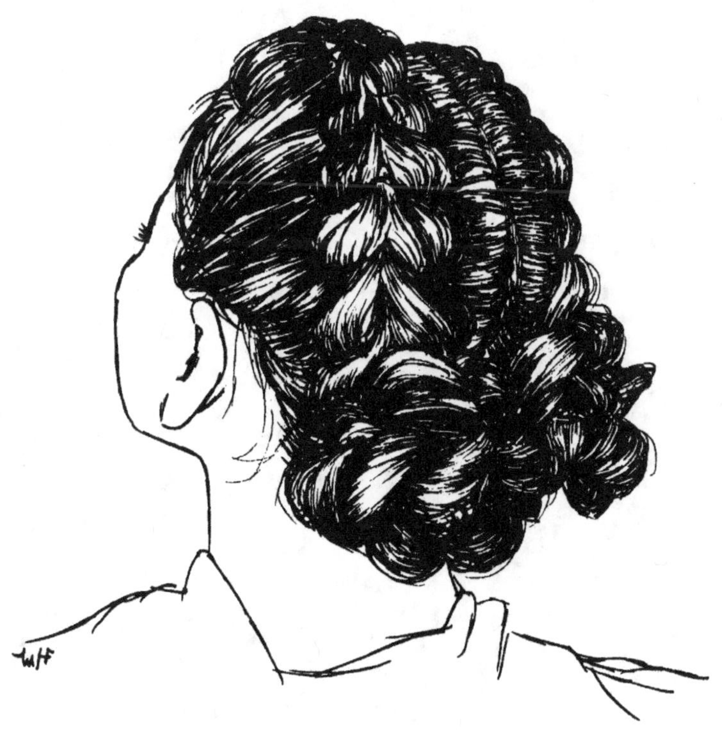

Erin Elizabeth

Pilocytic Astrocytoma Survivor

Erin

Hi! My name is Erin Elizabeth. I'm a full time graphics designer and part time fitness instructor. I am no hero, nor have I found a cure to save millions of lives. Honestly, I've lived a pretty normal and fortunate life. I am just a 28 year old girl who just had a little bit of bad luck. But hey, I'm alive and living an almost normal life, so who's to complain?

Life was being pretty good to me. Though the lens of my social media, @erinmurr it looked like I had a pretty perfect life, some would say. I was successful in my career, have the cutest puppy, hot boyfriend (he'll thank me for adding that) close supportive family and appeared to be extremely fit and healthy. I did everything to live a healthy life, I mean come on… I did whole30 twice. But what wasn't shared about my life was I was exhausted and I was never feeling well. I was moving so fast in life I never took the time to address how I really felt. I thought I was tired because I was so busy. I was working 50-60 hours a week in advertising, volunteering weekly at an animal shelter, picking up freelance design gigs for extra $, raising a puppy on my own (Milo; the best recovery snuggle buddy) teaching fitness 2x a week, sometimes more, attempting to get my blog off the ground, among keeping friendships alive and just living my day to day life. And don't get me wrong, this was the life I chose and loved, I was busy but I was happy. But then the dizziness, confusion, clumsiness, tingling in my arm and disconnected feeling of my legs struck. There became a point, my symptoms, I couldn't ignore anymore.

Spoiler alert; June 6, 2017 I was diagnosed with a brain tumor; later to discover it was a pilocytic astrocytoma, a pediatric tumor; meaning, I may have had it since adolescence. On scale of 1-4, 4 being most aggressive stage of cancer mine was a 1. There are many times I reflect on this and realize how lucky I am, my story could have been very, very different. But let me tell you my story, about how a normal girl like me blinked and her life was forever changed.

I had been symptomatic for months, possibly years, leading up to the surgery; for as long as I can remember I felt like this. I was struggling to remember what it felt like to truly feel well and healthy. I spent almost a year in and out of the doctors and ER (2 times) trying to figure out what was wrong. Every test showed I was the healthiest person in the room.

In the beginning it was the dizziness bringing me to my doctor, who first thought maybe it was a side effect to my heart burn medication. After a month of trying my medication at different times of the day or just not taking it, I realized that wasn't it and we went back to the drawing board. Professionals were then jumping to the conclusion that it was in my head; anxiety or I had an eating disorder. They had me journaling my food and drinking more water for possible dehydration.
Emotionally, this was taking a toll on me, I knew neither of these were the case but did as I was told to prove these theories wrong.

During this period of time (3-4 months) I was losing feeling in my left arm, weird tingly sensation or having out of body experiences when walking. It was as if I had to think how to walk; I couldn't feel my legs beneath me. But the dizziness was worsening. The room would get wonky all the time, as if I was in a fun house. Sometimes I would even have to grab something to stable myself. Not to mention these dizzy spells/fun house feelings, would hit me at the absolute worse times; teaching fitness, presenting work to clients or just out with friends. The dizziness was getting hard to ignore or write off as nothing. I was uncomfortable and couldn't figure out what was wrong but I knew this was NOT normal. Again doctors kept saying it might be anxiety... which at that point maybe it was, imagine going almost a year with the room becoming a fun house, you'd get anxious too.

It was a Thursday and I was on a conference call when the biggest "dizzy" spell hit me, I was sitting. I was starting to panic inside, why is this happening what's wrong with me. I couldn't focus and coworkers said I wasn't looking well. I left for home. I don't remember much of the walk home but grabbing everything I could to ground myself. I called my PCP who told me to go to immediate care (maybe it was some sort of flu/bug). I called my sister and boyfriend and said whoever can get to me first, I need help. I felt so unstable I couldn't stand. My boyfriend made it to me first and we went to the immediate care who then directed us to the ER.

Hours at the ER, yet again all the test were coming back healthy. I felt frustrated even going, having the feeling it was going to go the same as usual, tests would point to me being the healthiest person in the room... but not this time.

After several hours of heart, lung and blood tests a doctor had a mission to figure out what was wrong. This doctor, probably saved my life. He finally understood I wasn't a dramatic 27 year old. He looked at me and goes, you're uncomfortable, aren't you? I wanted to cry or scream but I nodded. He asked me to list anything and everything that was bothering me even if it was a scratch. I listed a few things and by luck I suppose, I had been having shoulder muscle pain. With that he ordered a CT scan of my neck to make sure I wasn't having mini strokes. A mini stroke?!? I thought to myself, how?!?   I'm 27. What would that mean for the future? The test came back negative. But there was something else, they saw a shadow. The scan for my neck picked up the shadow in my brain. At that point my parents were on their way and it was probably close to 4 am. They sent me back for a high contrast MRI which showed a mass, possibly a cyst in my cerebellum. Believe it or not they released me and I thought nothing of it. I was released with the instructions to see a neurosurgeon within 3-5 days. By then it was 6 am and a cyst seemed like something people treat daily and again I thought nothing of it.

The next day I didn't go to work since I hadn't slept but went along living life as normal. Monday came around. I was directing a photoshoot when I realized I forgot to call to schedule an appointment with a neurosurgeon. I called, for some reason still not realizing the severity. I was scheduled to see a surgeon the next day (by luck I would later find out he was one of the top surgeons in Chicago.)

Tuesday, June 6, 2017

I had my dad meet me at Northwestern Hospital, in Chicago for my visit. I arrived there first, took the elevator 22 flights up, and went to check in the neurology department. The lady kindly redirected me to the neurosurgeon side. **SURGEON**, it hit me, this was no checkup.

My dad arrived and we were taken back to a room (a room I one day pass out in when having my stitches taken out.) They did a bunch of funny tests to check my coordination. Touch your nose touch my finger, a test that would soon be difficult, and an hourly check. Walk in a straight line, balance, etc.

The doctor came in, who looked way too young to be a surgeon, I might add. But his bedside manner was by far the best. He talked with me for a little bit and ran a few more tests then got straight to it. He was direct and honest. Calmly, he said, "you have a tumor in your cerebellum" You could tell he'd had some practice delivering this news. My mind shut down and the room became silent in my head. I missed the next few minutes of him talking, I couldn't wrap my head around it. The silence broke, as my eyes swelled up with tears, I bit the inside of my lip so hard, trying to be strong and keep it together. I didn't want to admit to myself or anyone I was scared. Trying to hold back tears and stay strong. I fluttered my eyes dry and asked if I could see the scans. I didn't believe him. How?! How could this happen to me, I eat clean, I workout, I don't do drugs, I barely even drink. I do everything right to live a healthy life, so how could this be true?

Night and day. The MRI was night and day, big white circle like a full moon right there, couldn't have been clearer. He went over my options, explaining what my next year or more would entail. He went through the procedure and explained it'll be far worse before it gets better, which he might have undersold that statement. Recovery will be 12-18 months but can be longer. What's next, I asked?! Knowing my mind was made up, I knew I didn't have much of a choice. At this point we weren't sure if I had cancer or not. He told me I was to sleep on the information I was given and book the OR later in the week, knowing he would perform brain surgery to remove my tumor.

I sat in a chair in the main lobby as my dad made calls to my family. Still in shock, a million thoughts flooded my mind: how do I tell people, how do I tell work, what's going to happen? I tried, I tried really hard to think of other things but for the next chapter of my life this will be all I can ever think of. I would muddle to myself, you're going to be ok.

I got a second opinion from a neurosurgeon in NYC who gave me one option: brain surgery. The next day I booked the OR. Less than 3 weeks away, on June 26, 2017, I would return back to Northwestern Hospital for a four hour procedure to remove my tumor and under go the most challenging chapter of my life.

In a blink of an eye my life flipped upside down. My life didn't change forever on June 26, my life changed forever on June 6, the day of my diagnosis. Even now, I struggle to realize all that I've gone through. At times I even block it out but still live in the truth of it daily. There are still so many things I can't do, I still can't walk a straight line 8 months later and I can't live my busy, crazy life that I loved. Telling my story and creating awareness of brain tumors helps me live the life I am fortunate to still be living.

I tried, I really did. I tried crying but nothing really would come out. Sure my eyes would swell with tears now and then. It was usually when I walked to work and it would hit me or when I was sitting at my desk staring at a computer screen. In those times the shadow of fear, doubt and death would find me.

For the next few weeks I would surround myself with people, I didn't allow myself to be alone for any long length of time. One, I was nervous (of my health) if something would happen while I was alone and two, if

I was around people I wouldn't cry. I didn't want to be scared and if I cried I felt like I should be scared. Many cried when I told them, hugs and I'm so sorry. I became numb, I didn't have much emotion at all. Part of me believes I was in denial for most of it; I straight up didn't believe it. It's still hard for me to believe it to this day. I would just lift my chin up and reassure others it will be OK. Although at times I certainly felt like I was lying, but saying it out loud helped. Staying positive helped.

Friends near and far reached out. Some I never heard from again and others showed me what true friendship is. Leading up to surgery my old high school guidance counselor would pick me up and drive me all around Chicago just showing me where he grew up and fun facts about the city. He, a few years prior had brain surgery himself and knew what I was about to face. When he didn't hear from me every few days he'd call and check in or pick me up for Italian ice. Trying to keep me busy and optimistic. Through it all I tried to stay as positive as possible.

Avoid the shadows and stay in the light, the best advice I got during this time. The shadows are the what ifs and fear. There will be many times the shadows will corner you but you're stronger than them. I would remind myself, I am stronger than them. I would constantly say it out loud, I will be ok, sometimes I didn't believe myself but I would continue to say so. I became my own life coach, cheerleader and support system. I've got this, I can do it. Big inhale, big exhale.

The day before surgery my old guidance counselor picked me up at 7 am took me to Bahia temple, a place of worship that welcomes all beliefs. There was silence and I prayed. Give me strength, give me hope. My family, boyfriend, and his mom who flew in town all went to dinner that last night and we went bowling. One last fun family moment before my life would consist of an ICU, months of needing help to stand, walk, talk, eat, bathe, etc. And making a permanent indent on the couch in my childhood family room.

June 26, 2017

The day of surgery I arrived at 5 am with my parents for my high contrast MRI and testing prior to surgery. I didn't want to face or see anyone that morning. I left them all the night before with happy faces. The thought of seeing them before surgery made me feel as if it were good bye. And I couldn't let myself think that, it wasn't goodbye, was it?

The morning went quick, they didn't have me wait around very long at all. Hospital gown on, one of 5 IVs in. Reality of it all started sinking in. I had tags on my wrists for my blood type in case of an emergency. Signing please resuscitate papers, organs can be donated if something happens, etc. Sometimes I look back wondering how I had the strength to do it.

It was becoming real, brain surgery. The risk. A lot of risk, they told me chances of me walking on my own for months were slim and when I woke up I would need assistance and eventually a walker or cane. A tremor I could produce in my hand unseen to the untrained eye. Coordination will be challenged and relearned as for many other things I would have to rebuild strength to do.

Each person assisting came in to introduce themselves, senior surgical resident, nurses, surgeon and my team of 2 anesthesiologists. My anesthesiologists probably has no idea how he affected my life, but one day I must thank him (in addition to my ER doctor, I thank my surgeon every time I see him.) Anyways, my anesthesiologists asked if I wanted to be "knocked out" before they took me back to the OR, most people do he said but I said I wanted to see the OR (I regret that now). As they wheeled me out of the room barley able to say bye to my parents. My siblings, boyfriend and his mom came running down the hall as I was being taken away, (talk about dramatic.)

The OR was everything and more than I imagined, it's not like the TV shows. There was a scary contraption for my head to be stabilized in, metal with pins (or looked like that to me). The fear was setting in. I was cracking jokes and laughing nervously. I met my lead nurse who said she'd braid my hair back around where they would shave, to keep the area clean. They were all moving at a professional pace. My anesthesiologist talked to me again, preparing me for surgery. I think he could tell fear was all I had in my eyes. He put his hand on my arm and said "I promise you, you're going to be ok" and that's the last I remember. And for that I must thank him, because for the first time I truly believed it.

The week in the ICU was a blur, I remember bits and pieces. I remember them asking me my name, date, president etc. touch my nose touch their finger; hourly. I remember the nurses who got me through the week. I remember when the nurse hit the toilet and it cracked off the wall and the toilet was replaced completely in 20 min. I remember when my body when into shock and beeping of the machine went off. I remember the panic and all I wanted was to hold my parents' hands, for the fear of the unknown as the doctors were checking my heart for the concern of too much stress on it during surgery. My heart tests came back normal and I eventually fell asleep for the night…woken every few hours for tests.

I remember standing when they didn't think I could. Hooked to a big plastic belt for the physical therapist to hold and assist me with. I remember walking and my surgeon was as surprised as everyone else but extremely pleased; this was day 2. I couldn't talk, open my eyes or lay flat for weeks. But I listened, I listened a lot. The sacrifices my ICU nurses make to take care of me and others is incredible. I remember when they removed the drain out of my head, I remember they told me to go to a happy place such as Hawaii, a beach, somewhere warm and all I could think about was my childhood home, Simsbury, CT, siting on Talcott Mountain with my 4 best friends from childhood by my side and for a moment, I felt safe, that safe feeling of home. I remembered when they told me that the container clipped to me held my brain fluid and it didn't phase me. I remember the surgeon telling my family it was benign. I remember the tears and cheers of joy. I remembered the smile I gave, the same smile that had been lost through the journey.

Exceeding expectations, I was released to go home after a week in ICU, strong enough to skip the rehabilitation center, but still a long journey ahead with lots of self motivation.

I was the lucky one, I lived to tell my story.

The world spun around me, too dizzy to walk more than a few feet and too weak to pick anything up. Too scared to turn my head or move. I sat for weeks with my eyes shut, communicating by nodding. The steroids caused me to be over-heated then freezing cold all at the same time. I'd wake up in a sweat or stomach turning. Headaches became the norm, sometimes manageable and other times frightening. My walking was always supervised, everything was supervised, my mom became my full time nurse. Being sure I was given the correct medicine with food at the appropriate time, weening me off the steroids and pain killers.

I would track my steps with my Fitbit excited to get 200 steps in one day which was extremely difficult. I didn't want to get up but my dad would set a timer for every hour to go off to get me moving. My highlight of the day and goal was walking down the driveway each day to get the mail, wasn't even my mail. Milo (my 1 year old pup) stuck by my side and ever so gentle.

Sleeping was a challenge. I was unable to lay flat for some time, so you can imagine how hard it was to fall asleep. I had to have someone check my stitches and make sure no fluid was coming from them (lovely). All was healing well. My senses were heightened, I could hear things most people couldn't hear especially when I couldn't open my eyes (too sensitive to the light and enhanced the dizziness) I could hear music from my neighbor's house with TV on in my house. It was insane. I had to rely on my family and others greatly, to walk with me, feed me, set my shower up, (chair and towel because I couldn't stand on my own and the tub was too dangerous) I do remember my first shower, I was too nervous to touch my head or wash by the stitches. Someone was close by at all times, even when I used the bathroom, someone would have to stand outside. Most of this is a blur to me now. I was overwhelmed with emotion during this time, so grateful to be alive and able to walk without a walker (just a sway to my left) but I still hadn't cried, I didn't have the energy to cry, hell I couldn't open my eyes for it was too hard.

Two weeks post surgery I would return to see my surgeon, it was a difficult hour trip into the city and every bump in the road bothered me. Once I got there I had to walk inside 20 feet to then sit down to rally myself and tell myself I can do it, to make it to the elevator. I made it finally with my mom's help. I had my eyes closed for most of it. I remember checking in, looking around to see the waiting room full. My heart sunk into my stomach because I knew most if not all the people in there have or will have a similar story. I don't remember much more other than the nurse cutting some of my hair when removing the stitches (I already lost enough when they shaved 5 inches up). I then passed out on the nurse and eventually was told everything looked good and was free to go home. It had only been 2 weeks but I felt like I was getting worse, I had just finished my steroid treatment. The surgeon explained the steroid powered me through the past two weeks and now I've hit a wall and it's on me to rally and motivate myself to get better, for the steroid is not pushing me. I slept the whole ride home.

Three weeks post surgery, I was becoming less sensitive to noise and light and was able to start watching a little TV. Ellen quickly became a part of my routine. Three pm I watched Ellen and ate ice cream, I ate 10 pints in 7 days…with a little help. I was losing weight I didn't have to lose. My body burning so much energy to recover and muscle deteriorating from being stuck sitting, something my body was unfamiliar with. Ellen gave me something to look forward to and smile about each day. They were reruns, but I didn't mind. Few friends came to visit, I was not much of a host - being that there was nothing I could do but sit, sometimes just in silence. Most days it was just me and Milo, sitting there in silence. The get well cards were still flooding in.

The next 4-5 weeks were all pretty similar; learning how to walk further and with opposite hand with foot, something I had to think through in order to do. My big social outings were to physical therapy 2x a week. Eight weeks went by with lots of help from my family. I decided I was ready to return back to work and move back to the city (which I now have realized I was NOT ready). Returning back to work about one month too soon, I felt it. Barely making it through a day, exhausted, always with a headache and too much over stimulation. Awful tension headaches and more challenges than my body was capable of taking on. Each week was a struggle and most weekends I would crash and need to rest and sleep. Couldn't see my friends, go out, go out to dinner, etc. I became a hermit, luckily I had my boyfriend and dog by my side, so I wasn't entirely alone. But even with all of this going on, I somehow was able to stay positive and remember how lucky I was to be alive.

I was the lucky one…

A few months go by, still symptomatic, every few weeks it improves but then I add a new task to my routine and symptoms return. I struggle going into places with a lot of light or reflection, it enhances the dizziness. Long conversations, I would get lost in and lose my train of thought easily. Long conversations also take a lot of energy and by the end I could take a nap. I easily get sick with any and every cold. Started physical therapy with someone new in the city who had a neuro background and we began to strengthen VOR and balance. I can't walk in a straight line or turn my head too quickly without getting the fun house spins.

Frustration begins to kick in, feeling dizzy, sick, headaches and exhaustion. The emotional aspect is starting to catch up, I start wishing it had never happened and wondering why me. I wasn't feeling so lucky anymore. Lucky would be to never have had a brain tumor. It isn't fair, I want my old life back. I want to see my friends, go out, run errands without being scared, run a work meeting without getting lost in my head or too tired. I want to run, sprint, jump without my head hurting or my shoulders and neck to not be painfully stiff.

I'm currently moving into my 8th month post recovery. When I look back and see where I started, I can say I impress even myself. Most importantly I am ALIVE. I may have no feeling on part of my skull, lots of side effects and still cannot walk a straight line but I'm here for a reason I am alive to tell my story and help others navigate through this mentally and physically difficult journey and assure people they are not alone. In life sometimes it has to get worse before it gets better, but in time it truly does get better.

Even in the hardest, most frustrating times, I could shake it off and find that inner positivity and strength. Even when it was barely to be found, I would find it. People might have thought I was crazy, telling my story and being so positive and optimistic, but I am alive aren't I?

I am the lucky one. Jan 21, 2018 I lost one of the most beautiful, gracious and kind people in my life, my grandmother. An unexpected death, an undiagnosed brain tumor. Yes we had very different tumors and cases but it hit me harder than a bag of bricks how incredibly lucky I am that ER doctor took a risk on me and took one more test. I fought for myself, knowing something was not right. Who knows what my future would've brought. I feel guilt at times that my family was taken through this twice in less than 8 months. I know what my grandma was feeling and makes my heart sink, a realization hard for me to grasp and haunts me.

Again, I still have a long journey ahead and face lots of challenges and frustrations weekly wishing my life was normal/healthy again. We can't live wishing that bad things had never happened to us. We must take the misfortunes and find strength in them. See the life lessons and find the silver lining. I like to think this happened for a reason, I had the strength to overcome and now spread awareness and help others. I know what it's like and want to be that friend/support I needed. This experience, that most would consider awful, has introduced me to many amazing people who have also been challenged. These strangers have become my friends and my support system. Us survivors have the invisible sickness, most would never know just looking at us. Unless we tell, some if not all our symptoms are invisible to the strangers' eye.

This experience provides incredible perspective. You'll have a clearer vision of what's important in the world. The petty or materialistic things that bug you will fall by the wayside, and you'll just be really grateful to be alive. With that, the best thing you can do is to hold on to that feeling for as long as you can. Even as surgery becomes more distant in the rearview mirror and the obstacles become fewer, keep your newfound perspective, focus on the truly important things in life, and remember that every day is a gift—don't take that for granted. **I am a lucky one.**

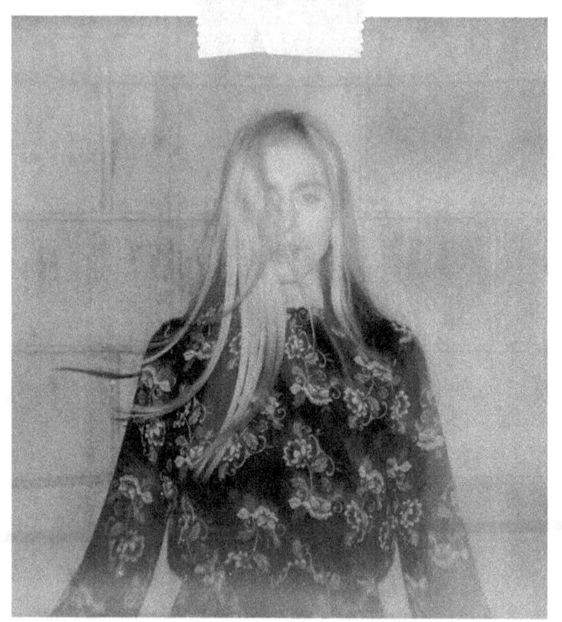

Minneapolis, MN

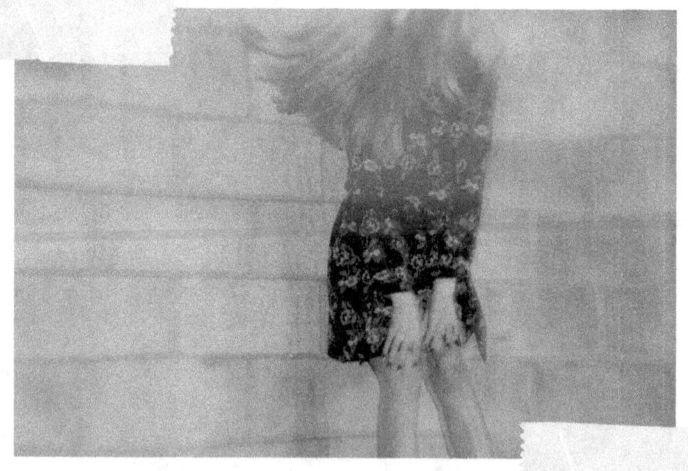

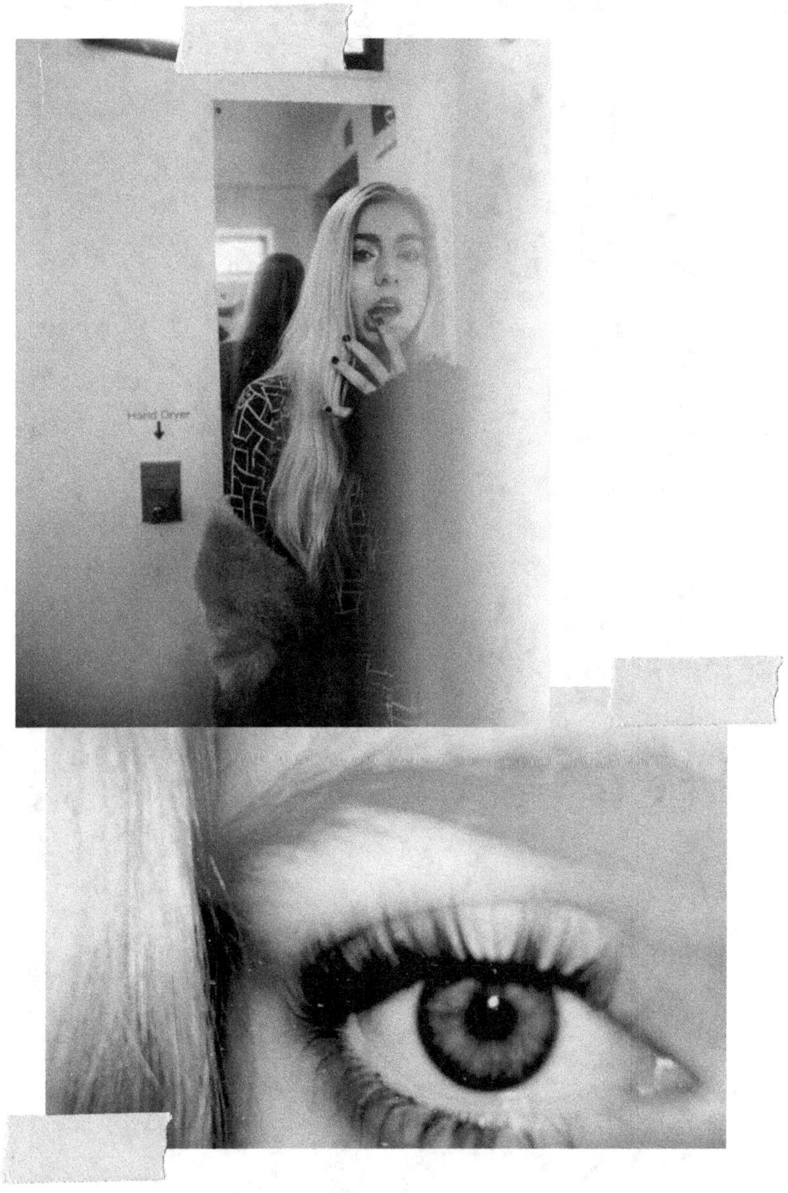

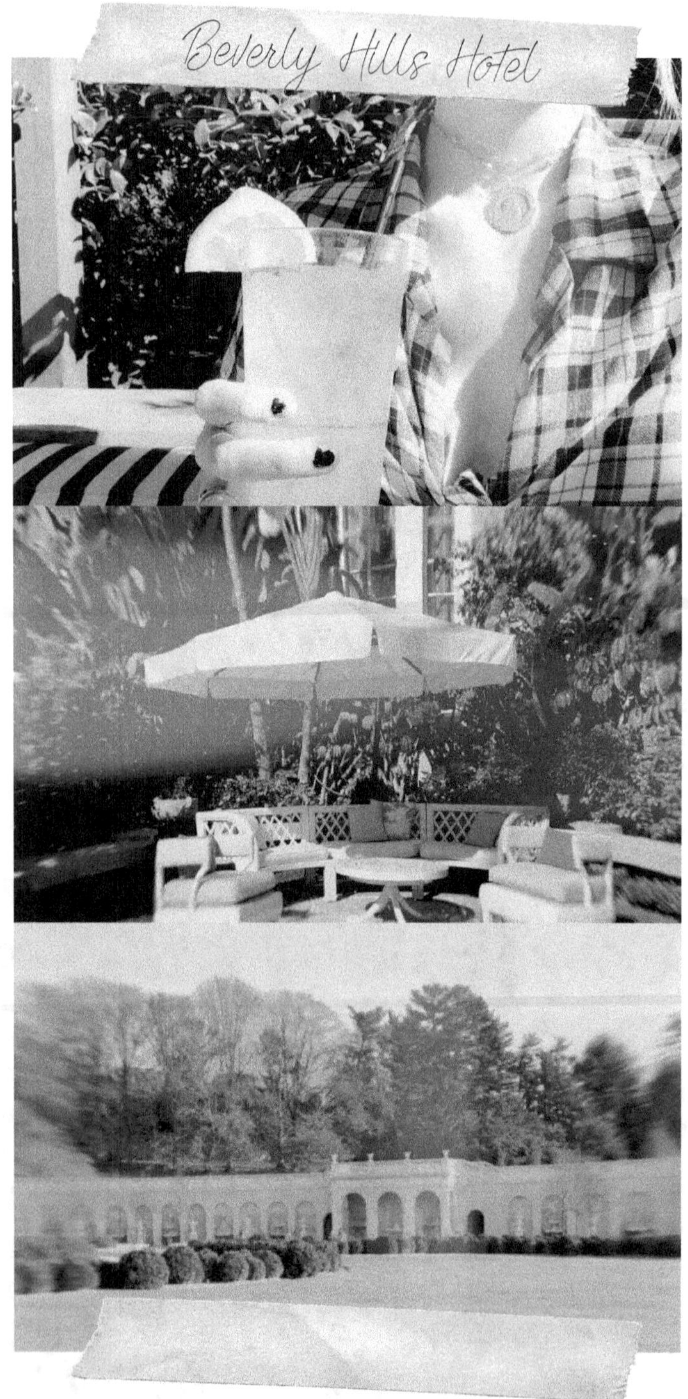
Beverly Hills Hotel

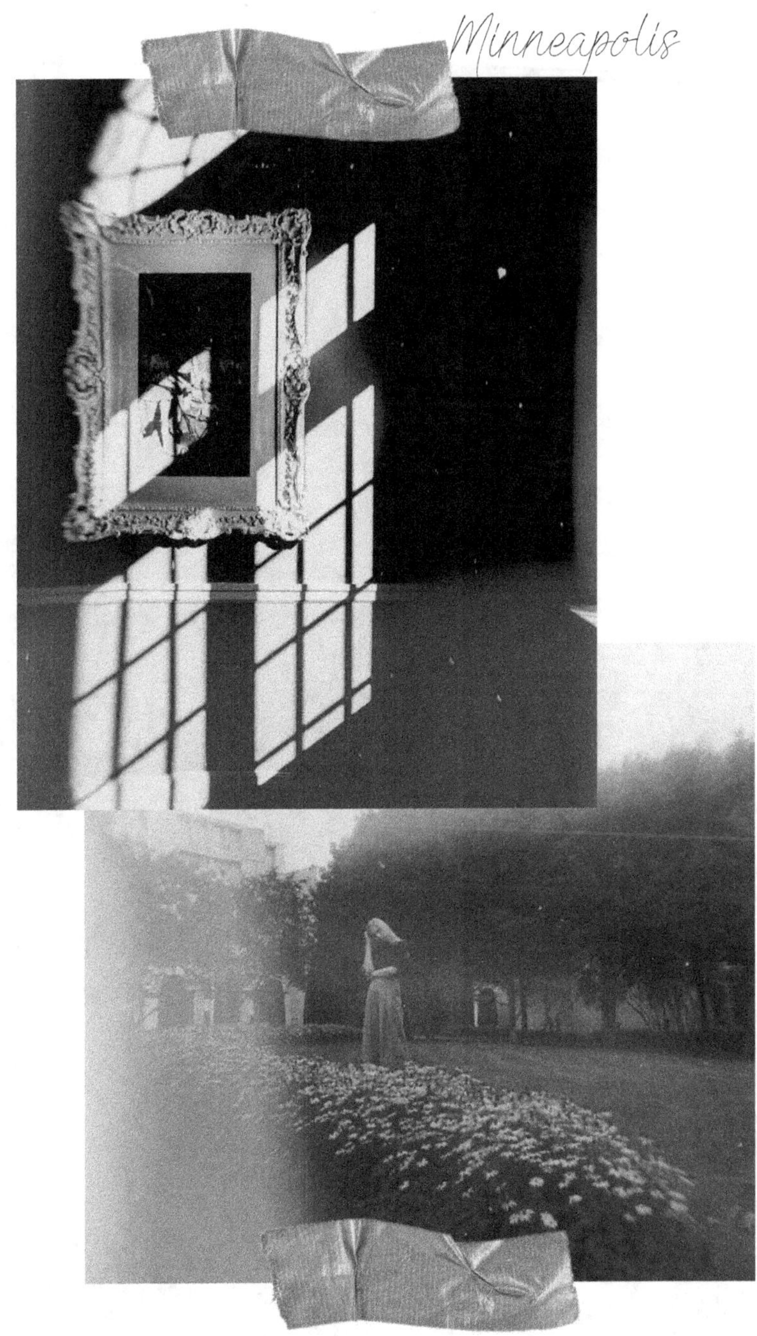
Minneapolis

Josh Perry

BMX Rider & Survivor

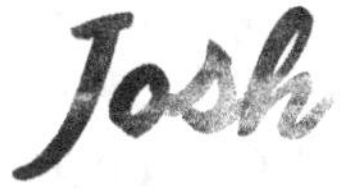

The Fall That Saved My Life

When you're younger people ask you what you want to become when you grow up. Many of us are asked this question but few make that dream a reality due to fear, not taking action, or going against our beliefs to fulfill someone else's dream- usually our parents.

I am one of few that can honestly say they made their dreams come true and still live that dream. One day that dream, and my life, were almost taken away from me. That is when I learned about what I believe are the most important shifts in my success to be a survivor rather than a victim. I don't just mean survivor as in living or dying, but I mean in how I show up in life and choose to participate. Too often I see people from all walks of life turn into a victim whether it be an injury or disease, didn't make the team, got laid off from a job, lost a game, failed a test, and so on. I choose not to look at things as failures anymore, rather learning opportunities. I call it "collecting data" for my next success.

The shifts I mentioned are as follows in no particular order: Perspective, Gratitude, a Vision (which equals goals & motivation), Visualization, and Health (Mindset, Nutrition, Fitness).

I believe I am successful in life because of these five shifts, a belief that anything is possible, the drive to get up and try again, and resilience to bounce back from any fall or failure. I also believe my immense passion for life is due to these shifts and have become strengthened with proper nutrition and fitness. I also believe any successful person has been conditioned by adversity to become strong and not give into fear. We also use "failures" as a learning opportunity rather than become crippled or paralyzed by it. At the end of the day, it's just a collection of information, and you choose how to use that information. You can choose to let an experience rob you of your hopes and dreams, or you can let an experience fuel your fire even higher. Some experiences may change your reality, and the path will be critiqued, but Gratitude, Perspective, and a Vision are the driving forces behind letting you slip into the victim seat.

My name is Josh Perry, and I'm a pro BMX athlete and a holistic brain health coach living with four brain tumors. But don't let the tumors fool you, I'm still thriving and progressing in all areas of my life, including my BMX and fitness training, businesses, and personal life. I use the tumors as a reminder to wake up grateful to be a living human and to foster a daily fire of motivation that keeps me going and going. Although I may come off a tad shy and quiet at first, my brain has a million things going on inside of it at all times, and once I feel comfortable, I can talk for days.

I was 17 when I moved 13 hours away from home on Cape Cod to Greenville, NC, dropping out of high school with my parents support, to ride and train with my idol, childhood hero, and mentor Dave Mirra. I quickly made a name for myself around the world from my videos, contests placings, style of riding, and inventing tricks, which won me a Harley one weekend. I found myself making friends with all my childhood heroes, being on national television programs, and riding X-Games! Then one day that all was threatened as I would learn my life was at risk unless I had open cranial surgery.

I fell during a routine BMX session and hit my head, regulating in a slight concussion. An MRI later and I would learn that fall saved my life. The doctor reported a brain tumor taking up the left half of my brain and that if I wanted any shot at riding again, let alone living, I would need surgery right away. I met with a surgeon at Duke University, and he said I was very lucky I fell when I did because if I didn't, he gave me a month or two until I may not wake up one day.

I hear people say I am "lucky," "it must be nice to do that" in regards to my career and lifestyle, or "that's got to be the worst thing to ever happen to you". I hear them non stop in regards to me, my life, and my story. None of it is true unless you decide to see it that way. I don't because it takes away the credit that goes to my mindset and choices over the years. Let me explain…

Let's start with **"You're lucky"**….am I? For which am I lucky? For my life that I worked harder for than most people are willing to, to create the life I dreamed of? Or for my choice to try a new trick that day out of a foam pit, resulting in a crash that saved my life? I see it not as luck for either, yet hard work, determination and choices. Had I not chosen that path in life, I may have never found the tumor and died in my sleep after suffering even longer than I had already suffered up to it being removed. Had I not worked my ass off for the life I desired and now live, I would find myself in the shoes of the person saying **"you're lucky"** to live that life. **Luck had nothing to do with it, it was**

all due to taking action, a belief, and never giving up.

Now, what about "it must be nice" in regards to my lifestyle as a pro athlete with no "real job". Haha, this couldn't be further from the truth as I bust my ass day in and out and have done so since I was 13 to make my reality manifest into what it is, and continue to do so. "It must be nice" is a cop-out, in my eyes, to taking a risk for what you truly want in life and settling for the status quo. A "real job" is defined as being unhappy, a slave to time and money, stressed out and feeling unfulfilled in your life. I have supported myself since I was 17 and decided to move away from my parents to follow a dream. I would say doing what I did/do to be able to pay my bills qualifies as a real job and it is so great to say that. It must be nice because it truly is. Anyone who says "it must be nice" has the same opportunity to live the life they dream of. All it takes is the belief that change is possible and the determination to take action and not give up.

Finally, "that's got to be the worse than to ever happen to you". I did see it that way while dealing with a diagnosis, surgeries, recovery, etc. Then one day it clicked as I reflected on gratitude for being alive and still riding my bike. That experience led me to changes my ways of living on so many levels to become the healthiest, happiest, strongest and most successful I have ever been while just progressing more and more. It's led me to sharing my story and inspiring people around the world thanks to my BMX career, learning about proper health and sharing that with others, which is now a business of mine, starting a charity to give back to those in their biggest times of need like I once was, and so many other great changes in my life. It's in turn the greatest thing to ever happen to me and I am grateful for that first diagnosis and surgery, the second diagnosis and Gamma Knife Radiosurgery and the two tumors shrinking, and the third time, which resulted in a massive shift with my health to the point a year later with no treatment the 2 new tumors have stalled in growth and I am still 100% with my life.

The point of my story is that life is all a matter of perspective and choices. We can choose to see the world as evil, play the victim card, and think life happens to us. Or, which I prefer, we can choose to see the world as beautiful and full of opportunity, see that there is no failure but just learning opportunities, see that life happens for us, know we can do whatever we believe we can do, and choose to be a **survivor** when times get tough, which all leads to success, love and happiness.

176

Meghan Pawlak

Cyst On Pineal Gland Survivor

Meghan

I have repeated what type of tumor I had,

why the doctors didn't believe me,

that yes I'm okay (now),

and thank you for your kind wishes

so many times, it's become a script.

I have become detached
whenever I talk about it.

I'm on autopilot,

but it still kinda hurts.

Moving on is all I've wanted to do since the day I found out I was having brain surgery. My friends and family asked me why I would write about it if all I wanted to do is move on. This time I'm not going to go off my script.

I'm going to write about me,

                              not my tumor,

my experience,

                              not statistics,

        and how I became a survivor.

I was 12 and I had horrible symptoms, mainly a constant headache, when I found out I had a cyst on my Pineal Gland. There was only one doctor in the country who would do surgery on it, and he lived in Houston. We found him online because the doctors at home were leading us down a path of pills that just made things worse. When we got to Houston for the consultation he said he would do the surgery as soon as possible. If not I would've been blind and in a wheelchair within a couple years.

When we went down back down to Houston for the surgery we planned on staying for a month in case anything happened while I was recovering. We drove down from New York and got to stop in New Orleans, which was amazing. We did a lot in Houston and it was great spending time with my parents.

I had the surgery on October 26th, my Nana's birthday. After the surgery I called her to wish her a happy birthday, she was so happy she cried. I was only in the hospital for three days, then I went back to the hotel.

The first week of recovery was the worst week of my life. I couldn't hold anything down and I couldn't watch TV or read; I just had to lay down and rest. I could barely sleep at night and when I could, my mom would have to wake me up to take pills.

After about two weeks I was doing a lot better. We ended up leaving early because of how well I was doing.

I had a lot of support from everybody in my neighborhood. Everyone really helped out. I didn't love the attention I was getting but I loved the kindness of all these people I didn't know.

It was weird going back to school because I was starting high school so I was the new kid. I hadn't seen my friends in forever because I had isolated myself. They all lived on while I was on pause and it was hard readjusting.

Today, over a year past the surgery I'm doing so much better. There are still bumps in the road here and there but I've learned that it's a long recovery process. I am so grateful for the support and generosity from everybody and how much I've grown.

Party Next Door

there's a party next door
on the fifth floor
i'd like if you come
it might be fun
i don't know it's just a thought

there was a party yesterday
but you had to pay to get in
it reminds me of when...
I don't know it's just a thought

there's a party next month
and I think they invited a bunch
of your friends
it reminds me of when...
I don't know it's a just a thought

there's a party next door
on the fifth floor
i'd like if you come
it might be fun
i don't know it's just a thought

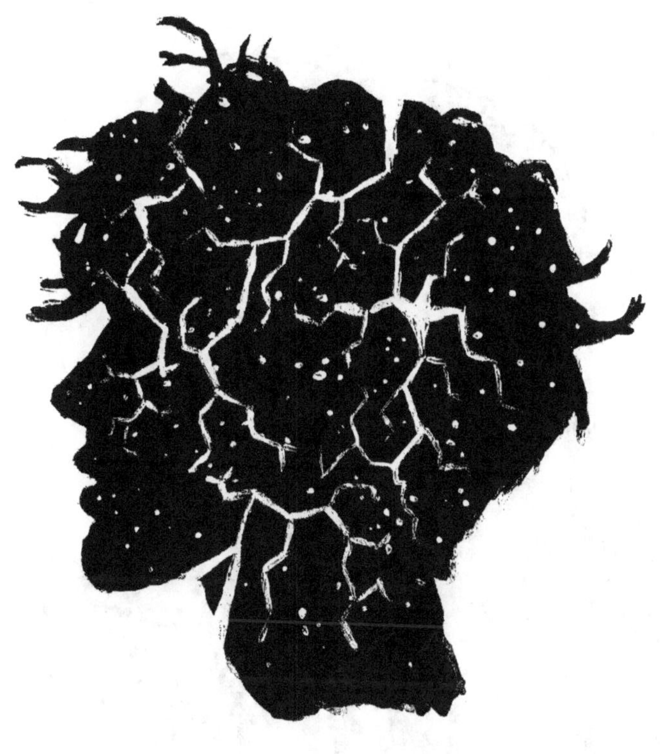

Sketch By Maryline Platevoet

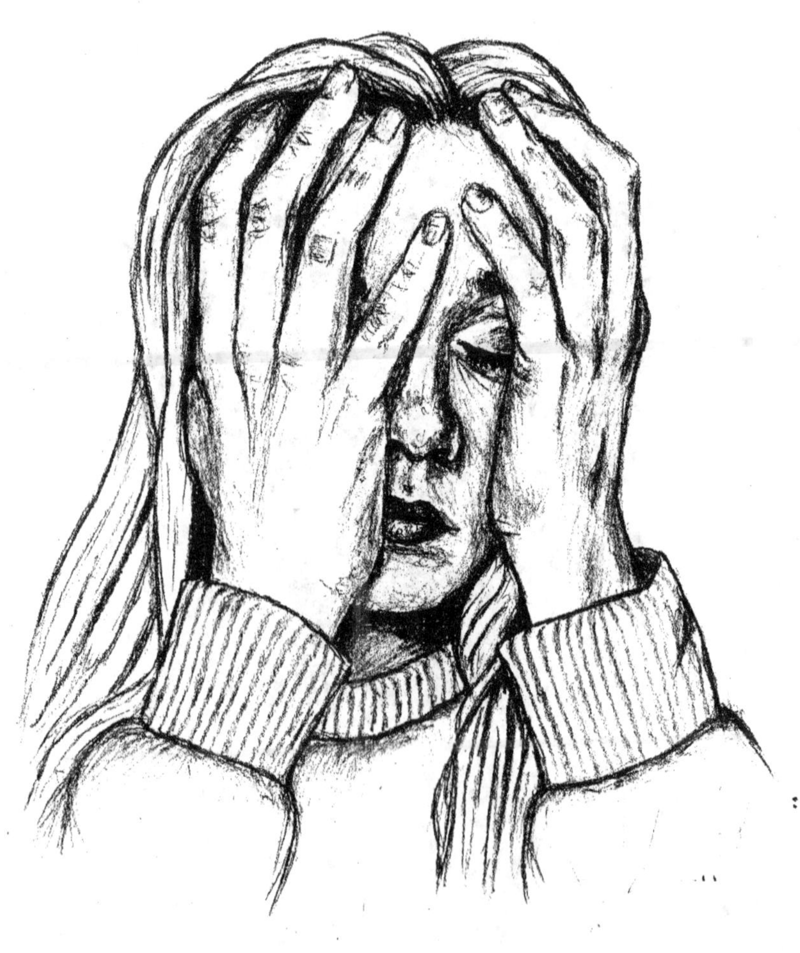

Sketch By Maryline Platevoet

STRANGER

never met this lady before
but I'm crying on her kitchen floor

everything is coming too soon
now I'm crying on her sofa in the
living room

never even been here before
but I'm crying on the bathroom floor

I blink
and I open my eyes too soon
now I'm crying on the table in the
dining room

been here a while
it's half past noon
now I'm crying on the rug in the
bedroom

and for the first time in a long time…

she laughed.

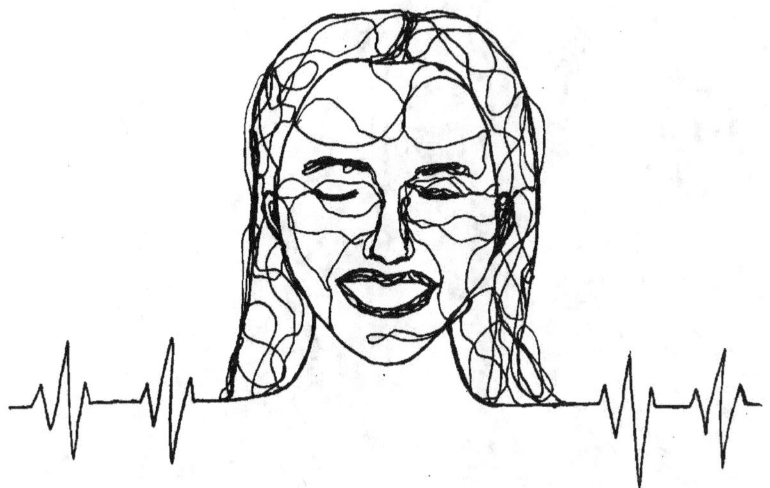

Sketch By Maryline Platevoet

New York City

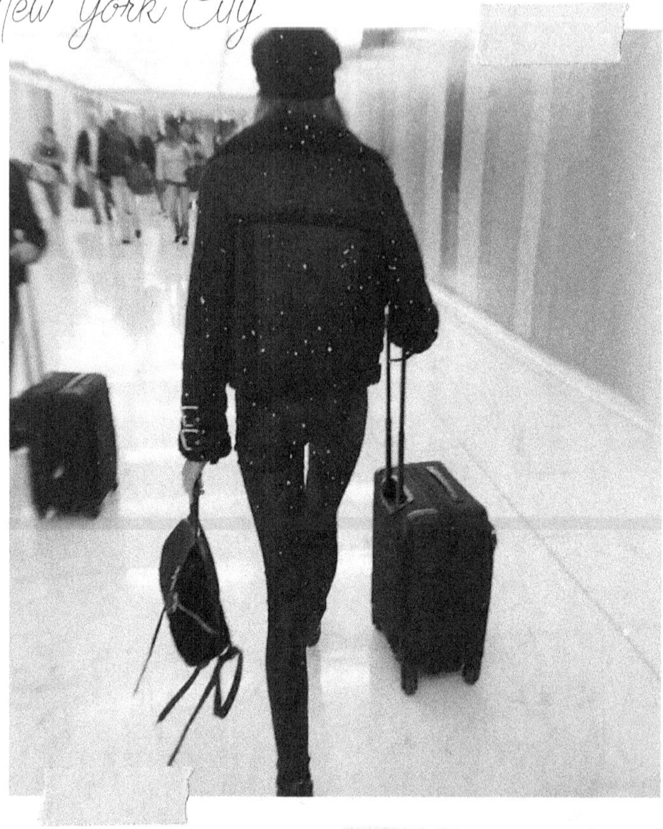

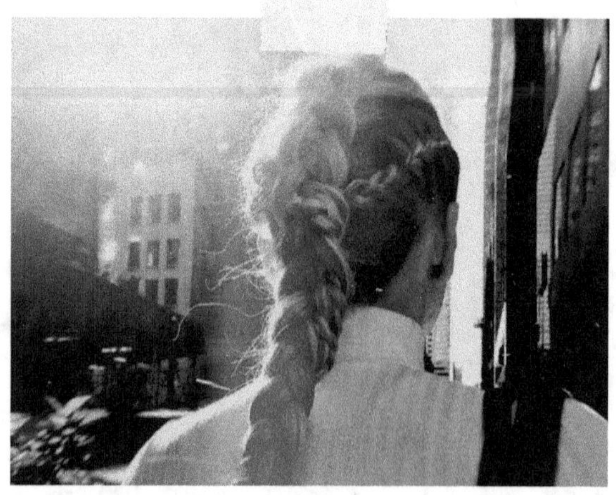

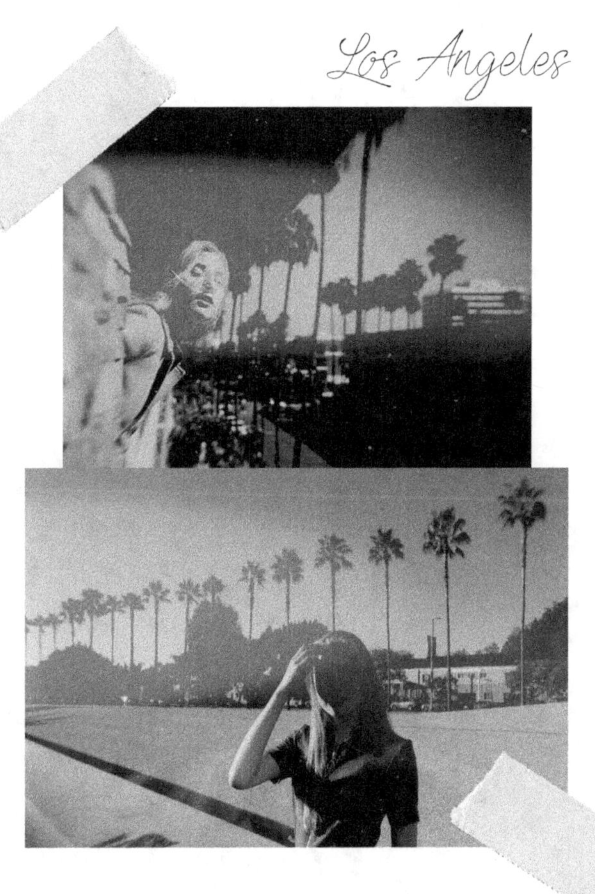
Los Angeles

Suzanne Turpie

Mother Of Medulloblastoma Survivor - Caleb

Suzanne

September 4th, 2015 will be forever etched in our minds as the day our life changed. It's the day that my son lost all innocence. It's the day that our life fell apart and the day that made everything change forever.

Caleb was 9 at the time. He'd been sick for around 6 weeks. He had vomiting some mornings and sometimes quite severe headaches. He looked pale and was just not his normal self. Our amazing doctor (Sandy Clarke) ran countless tests, with one coming back that he had a stomach bug. This was treated with antibiotics and we were hopeful that this was the cause and he'd be all fixed up after 10 days of treatment, but we were wrong.

We questioned his school about any potential issues but were confident that there were none. Caleb was a well-liked individual at school and we didn't think there was anything wrong on the school front, but we were clutching at straws trying to get to the bottom of Caleb's illness.

Our doctor then organized for a quick appointment to be made with our local pediatrician.

When we saw him, Dr Johnson did a couple of neurological tests and noticed that Caleb had a slight tremor in his hand and was unable to walk heel to toe in a straight line. He organized for an MRI to be done.

Leading up to the MRI, I started to notice that Caleb was forgetting things he should know or has known for years. In my head, I had alarm bells ringing.

On the day of the MRI, I took the day off work and took Caleb to the appointment. He had his scan done and we were given the pictures on a disc and sent home. About an hour later I received a call on my mobile. It was a doctor from the hospital telling me I needed to come straight back to the hospital and to bring Caleb.

Upon walking through the doors at the children's ward, the doctor asked the nurses where she could go to speak to us. Their reply: "We are going to put him in bed six, so you can talk to them in there, as it's a private room." We were already frantic but this was proof that there was something seriously wrong with our boy.

Caleb was asked to go to the playroom and my husband Rob and I were sat down. The doctor calmly explained to us that they had found a tumor in the back of Caleb's brain and that he needed to be flown to Sydney, Australia. They were in contact with Sydney Children's Hospital and were finding out if they needed to start chemo straight away. We broke down and cried. We were terrified and absolutely shattered.

Caleb was bought in and the doctor sat him down and explained that he had something called cancer. Unfortunately for Caleb, he understood what this means. Only a short 16 months ago, our family had suffered the devastating loss of Caleb's 14-year-old cousin who lost her short battle to cancer. Caleb went into shock as for him, in his head, he thought this would mean that he was also going to die and never see us again.

Consoling Caleb was so hard. I soon learned how to put a smile on my face, even when inside I was breaking, and I learned how to hold back tears when inside I was losing it.

We started to make phone calls at this stage to notify everyone. I rang work and advised them that I would not be in…. This was the first encounter I had where I learned people just don't get it. I was told "now don't stress, I'm a mum too so I understand." I've learned since then how much I hate being patronized by being told things like this. None of it helps and you don't understand unless this has happened to you.

I remember so clearly getting dinner that night. I was standing out the front of a takeaway shop and I was breaking. I was watching people go about their normal life knowing that mine was full of uncertainty and despair.

The next morning Caleb and I were flown to Sydney. I was absolutely terrified and alone but I had to put my brave face on for Caleb and be as upbeat as possible. This was his first plane flight and he didn't mind it – he was pretty excited to be wheeled in a bed to a car, to then be driven to the airport. My husband Rob was making his way down by car. I can't imagine what that car ride by himself was like.

We were soon settled into a ward and it was there that things became quite hectic and have never really stopped. A surgeon and many doctors came around to discuss what would happen next. Caleb was scheduled for surgery on September 8th, 2015 and in the lead up to this day we just tried to keep Caleb's spirits high.

Surgery day was really hard. We had organized for Caleb's older brothers to have a 'fun' day in the city so they weren't around to see our anxiety or worry. I went with Caleb while they put him to sleep. I put my brave face on and I held his hand and I smiled with him and I joked with him and I told him how much I loved him. I told him I'd see him soon. What I'd do to go back to this moment and take one last long look at his smile.

Caleb was in surgery for around seven hours and when he came out into recovery we were told that they'd got most of the tumor but there was a small bit left and they were hopeful this would go with radiation.

We weren't prepared for Caleb in ICU. He was hooked up to a lot of machines and not responsive. I just sat there and held his hand and cried for my little boy. No child should ever go through that. I was unable to stay with Caleb that night in ICU as there was no room. This is the only night I didn't stay with Caleb in hospital.

We started to realize early on that Caleb wasn't 'ok' and that he had a 'droop' on the right-hand side of his face. We were reassured this was probably just swelling from surgery and it should subside, but it never did. Caleb lost all movement in the right-hand side of his face, he lost his beautiful smile. He was unable to sit, stand, or walk. In the coming months he would need a lot of rehab to be able to do this all again. In the meantime, Caleb didn't talk much and was in a wheelchair. He was completely dependent on us.

Official results came back which confirmed Caleb had brain cancer, medulloblastoma, and the next stage of treatment was discussed. This involved 6 weeks of radiation 5 days a week followed by 7 months of chemotherapy. We would need to live in Sydney – 5 hours from home. Away from my husband and our other 4 children.

Radiation was not fun and everyday was torture for Caleb. Having his head, face down, screwed to a table was extremely unpleasant and getting Caleb to cooperate to do this was hell. I would have done anything to trade places with him. I was able to talk to him through a microphone and watch him on a monitor, but I couldn't hold his hand.

You ever wonder how broken you can get when you're already broken?

Chemotherapy was also a very unpleasant experience. It made Caleb extremely sick and he lost a great deal of weight. A feeding tube was inserted early on as Caleb stopped eating. We hated every second of having a feeding tube. Caleb became very withdrawn and distressed. His mental state was very concerning. Caleb was very weak and still relied on a wheelchair, though he could now sit unaided and take steps with help.

We were fortunate enough that between chemotherapy, we could come back home to Port Macquarie for around two weeks. Getting to go home for these short periods of time was soothing to our soul. Sydney represents hospital and isolation, so it was nice to get out of there when we could.

In July of 2016, we were finally able to ring the cancer bell that signifies the end of treatment. This was a very emotional day. We went out for dinner that night to celebrate and prepared to head home.

What no one prepares you for is the life after cancer. For us life after cancer has been really hard. Caleb still continues to feel the effects of his treatment and requires further surgery to help get movement back in his face. He can walk unaided now. However for far distances he still uses a wheelchair. He is susceptible to any illness going around and gets sick very easily. He has OT, physio and hydrotherapy once a week on different days.

We don't really have any friends anymore. I guess while our life was on hold, everyone else's wasn't, and they moved on. We also found out that during treatment, a lot of people want something to do with you, as they get something out of it for themselves. Though they meant well and did really have our best interests at heart, it hurts a lot when after treatment, those people pretty much want nothing to do with you as there is nothing further in it for them. This is a harsh truth and one that I struggle to get my head around.

People don't really want to talk to you. They are scared they will say the wrong thing. It's extremely isolating this world that we live in.

Financially we've been hit pretty hard. I've not been able to return to work and we have added expenses with having to travel to Sydney frequently for check-ups. Life is pretty hard week to week but it's just something we need to get used to as I'm unable to return to work anytime soon.

Caleb is doing amazing things. He has been chosen as a school captain for 2018 which is simply amazing! The school community has truly embraced Caleb and loved and supported him unconditionally. Seeing Caleb be given a chance to be a child is so humbling.

On February 2nd, 2018, he was one of the Queen's Baton Relay runners for the Commonwealth Games. We travelled to Kempsey (an hour north of home) and with so much pride and emotion we watched Caleb carry the Queen's Baton. This was to go down in history as one of my favorite days ever with Caleb.

We've tried so hard to keep Caleb doing "normal" things and including him in all that we do. We try not to let him having a disability hold him back. We've enrolled him in karate, he did soccer, he loves swimming.

However, we are literally in a bubble, a huge cancer bubble. We desperately need funding for brain cancers so that my son Caleb can be given a complete chance at life. The statistics are so cruel to look at. Even though Caleb is doing so well, the statistics are only two in every ten people diagnosed with brain cancer will live five years or more after diagnosis.

Imagine needing funding for your child to have a chance at survival but there's not enough for it. Imagine knowing that if this cancer doesn't kill your child, that the treatment that "saves" his life could also destroy his life and ultimately take it also.

Maybe I should do more of a good job of sugar coating the reality of brain cancer and friends and real life, but I struggle so much with doing this. Life does suck, I'd do anything in heartbeat to take this away from my precious boy. Our life is permanently changed, and not in a good way. All our hopes and dreams are out the window – being able to renovate our house is just a dream (we bought a house that needed doing up and will remain this way for a long time now,) me being able to return to work is a faraway dream, updating cars; all those things that you usually plan. We try not to plan anything as things can change all too easily in the blink of an eye. In saying this though, we try to make as many memories as we can with Caleb and our kids now. We will do anything in our power to take them away on a short holiday, weekend away, camp trip, day trip as we feel this is so important in our life. We want to give Caleb a purpose to keep on living, to keep on fighting. Teach him that there is beauty in life despite what life has given him. We want to give him hope every single day. Without hope, we have nothing.

There’s a saying I love…

“Some people never meet their hero – I gave birth to mine.”

Kelsey Taveira

Mixed Grade II Oligoastrocytoma & Grade III
Anaplastic Astrocytoma Survivor

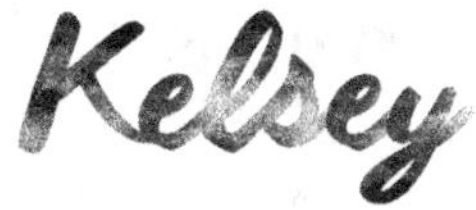

Kelsey's Journey

Hello! I am Kelsey Taveira. Born October 11, 1985 in Redondo Beach, CA. Thus far my life has been great! I am blessed with an amazing mom, dad and younger sister. My parents taught my sister and I the value of hard work, dedication, kindness and the importance of traveling. I went to school in Redondo Beach until college where I decided it was time to explore and find out what this beautiful world has to offer. I studied abroad in Salamanca, Spain and then Oxford, England from the ages of 19-20. It was 100% the best experience of my life and if you are reading this, I recommend studying abroad for you or someone you know. It has made me the person I am today.

After that, I continued my education at UNLV where I graduated with a Bachelors Degree in Event Management and Food and Beverage. After graduating I left Las Vegas and moved back to California where I had tons of amazing jobs in the event planning industry, including starting my own company. I ended up leaving the industry in 2013 and started as an independent brand partner with a holistic anti-aging company Nerium International. The experience ended up changing my life for the best and what I never imagined could happen. I have been able to work from anywhere at any time and finally felt at ease. I created financial freedom and time for myself which led to a lot of travel not just for work but for personal experience. It has also been the biggest blessing these past two years, I got to continue to work from home while in recovery.

My last big trip was to Thailand in December 2015 with one of my friends, Alison. We traveled the country for three weeks and ended with a yacht charter over NYE into 2016. Little did I know that charter would turn into the best week of my life and meeting my now husband. Fast forward to 2018, I am married to the captain of that charter in Thailand, Philip Taveira. We got married in our part time home Portimao, Portugal on September 2, 2017 with 112 of our friends and family from all around the world.

Life was good….but it still is. I WILL NOT let a brain tumor determine my happiness and future.

I discovered my brain tumor a week after returning from Thailand in January 2016 and went in for surgery days after. Philip flew to be by my side the day before surgery. The last two years I continued on my life like nothing really happened. I feel I was left in the dark about my diagnosis. The surgeon and doctors made me feel as if they removed the tumor and I was good to recover and then move on with life, like I did. I was referred to an oncologist at UCLA and the past two years have been following up there every three months with MRIs and 1 PET scan. I was "stable" at every appointment and "looked good" so why would I question that….good is good so I kept on with life.

Fast forward to November 16, 2017 where my MRI came back positive for regrowth and not just a regrowth, a growth of a tumor bigger then the size of when I began this journey almost two years ago. WHAT!?!?!? HOW in the world, in two years, was this tumor never noticeably growing on the MRIs? I was left with my un-detailed biopsy from the day after surgery and felt it was a tumor that was removed and was gone and I move along. Little did I know (now I know from my own research) that the type of tumor I have, a mixed grade 2 Oligoastrocytoma WILL grow back. It is only a matter of time.

So WOW! Here we are almost exactly two years later and I am faced with a regrowth of my tumor. My only option because of the size and type of tumor was another surgery. I had my second surgery on Jan 23rd with Dr. Linda Liau at UCLA. This time everything will be different. I not only have a whole new view on life but on how to live life. It wasn't until the tumor recurred that I feel my "journey with brain cancer" really began. So here I am, ready to not only to share my journey but to hopefully help prevent misdiagnosis and be an example of what to do when diagnosed with a brain tumor, cancer or other diseases. This is me, this is my story.

The Day It All Began

What started out as a normal night with a friend at dinner in Venice, CA turned in to a future I never expected. Just after ordering our food I started to feel dizzy, nauseous and confused. I have a history of headaches and anxiety so just thought I was maybe dehydrated or about to have a panic attack. The next thing I remember is waking up in the UCLA ER confused surrounded by my mom and dad. I had suffered a grand mal seizure outside of the restaurant and was rushed by ambulance to the ER. There, I had a CT Scan and the doctor determined there was a mass growing on the right side of my brain. The only words I could think to say was….what? I needed a MRI done but was given the ok to go home rest a little and go to the hospital closest to my home the next morning. After my MRI I found out I did in fact have a brain tumor and it was a size that would need removal ASAP. I ended up staying in the hospital and was monitored for a few days. Then I went in for the craniotomy. The surgery was six hours and the post-op pain was excruciating. I stayed in the ICU for two days and then recovered back in my original room for another two days until I was released to go home. My stay at Torrance Memorial was a long 11 days but I felt lucky, loved and had hope for a healthy promising future.

Planning For The Future & My Second Surgery

First came love, then came marriage, then we were ready to talk about the baby in the baby carriage. I found out about my brain tumor before we got married but my husband Philip was with me from the time I found out. There was no surprise that my tumor would be a huge part of our life and future planning. Of course we had the hope the tumor would never come back but the reality of that was untrue. Here we are after my second craniotomy still extremely optimistic and positive for a bright and beautiful future. We both love kids and always talked about not waiting too long to start a family. I LOVE kids so much and want my own badly. I feel so lucky to have accomplished so much in my life but truly feel the thing missing is me becoming a mother. I already am aware I am a high risk pregnancy case because of my tumor. I am also at a high risk for a lot of things that can happen during pregnancy like blood clots, tumor regrowth, the anti seizure medication I am on possibly being passed along to the baby. None of these are guaranteed but it still weighs on my mind.

Since all my past two year MRI scans had remained stable, we went in to the appointment on November 16, 2017 with excitement and confidence that my MRI was going to come back clear and we would be able to start discussing the possibility of starting our family. Well, that news changed FAST and I was left with the sad unbelievable news that pregnancy was not an option right now as my tumor was showing positive for regrowth.

At first my doctor mentioned I could possibly start treatments of chemo and radiation to try and shrink the tumor but later found out first I would need another surgery to remove as much of the tumor as possible and then we would determine the necessary future treatments. My doctor also told us that if we were that serious about starting a family and having our own children we should look into freezing our embryos to assure we would one day be able to. Chemo and radiation is so harmful to the body it would destroy all my eggs and chances of conceiving naturally. We sat on it for a day and weighed all the pros and cons. Cost was a huge concern as this treatment is extremely costly and sadly insurance does not cover ANY OF IT. It is so unfair and should be changed to help those like me that need it for a valid reason! After realizing the only real con was extreme costs, Philip and I decided it was worth it and we emptied our bank account which was also all our wedding gifts and honeymoon funds and decided to put all of that to this process. So if you are reading this and happened to have given us a wedding present or contributed to our honeymoon fund thank you because you were part of making this possible!! Instead of a honeymoon we got potential future children. And when the day comes and we have kids, you will be partly responsible for these little Parigian/Taveira rug rats running around! haha! So huge thank you!!!!!!! :) If you have additional questions for me on the actual process, procedure, anything really, I am more than happy to answer any and all of them but long story short, we ended up with 8 healthy embryos that are now frozen in the clinic.

Where I Am Today - After My Second Craniotomy

Overall everything went well! My biopsy and future treatments…not exactly what I expected. But are they ever…really?! Good news is the surgery was a success. I am here safe and sound, recovering well with little to no pain, had no changes in any of my cognitive functions and I'm feeling good.

I did have a set back when coming home after four nights in the hospital and experienced excruciating unbearable pain. I listened to my body and knew something was wrong. We went back to the UCLA ER and thank god I did because they discovered I had gotten a blood clot in the back of my brain and needed to start treating it ASAP. I stayed another four days in the hospital on a heparin drip until my blood flow opened up and left with a plan of twice a day Enoxaparin Sodium stomach injections. These will continue until the clot is fully dissolved which can take months to years. Hoping for the months. Also, a goal is to transition from the injections to a pill form.

They determined the cause was a mix of the brain tumor, surgery, being female, and recently being given a large amount of hormones from the IVF I had done the month before surgery. So that sucks, but I am grateful I found it and that I did the IVF for the future family we are planning on starting as soon as I am given the OK!   Now, for the craniotomy, Dr. Linda Liau is positive she removed close to 85% of the tumor. Considering it was the size of a large lemon (7cmx2.5cm) 85% is a large portion and since a tumor can never be 100% removed, 85% is considered extremely good news! My tumor was cut into 4 pieces, biopsied and kept in the neurology lab freezer at UCLA. I specifically asked to have it frozen for the reason that if needed one day, I can use it possibly for treatments that Dr. Liau is researching and soon starting trials for. I also gave them the OK to use some of it for research purposes. Another great thing about UCLA is all the research they do and that's why I chose to do my surgery there.

Now for the biopsy details. If you know nothing about tumors then this part will probably be like reading a different language. However if you do know about tumors, then you will understand how the change of tumor happened and that it is very common for a tumor to change grade and type over time. My first diagnosis in January 2016 after surgery was a Grade II Oligodendroglioma it then changed to a Grade II mixed Oligoastrocytoma about a year later. For the past almost 1.5 years it has remained as a Grade II mixed Oligoastrocytoma. This type of tumor at the time was benign and slow growing and didn't seem to act very positively to chemo and radiation. Because of this, I did nothing but follow up MRIs every three months like the Dr.'s told me to do.

If I knew what I do now, that the tumor was still there and had a 90% chance of growing back and would eventually grow back, then I would have of course started everything and anything holistic to try and prevent this monster from growing back. Which it did quicker than I ever imagined it would. To say I was and still am livid that I was not given proper information on my future with a brain tumor is an understatement, but I have decided to stop dwelling on the past and move on to the now.

Currently my diagnosis and tumor has changed. I now have a Grade III Anaplastic Astrocytoma, commonly referred to as an AA3. Although the change, it is still considered slow growing, so that is positive. Another positive is that the entire tumor is not grade III. It showed enough cells were grade III because of the tumor type changing to a full Astrocytoma; that is the reason for the updated diagnosis. I am also positive for the IGH1 mutation, 1p19q deletion, MGMT mutation and KI67 which is really good to have and also means the tumor will respond extremely well to the treatments of radiation and chemotherapy. So with all this news and meeting with my new NeuroOncology team at UCLA I have decided to move forward with the treatments of radiation and chemo. I begin Monday, March 12. Radiation is six weeks long Monday through Friday. I begin chemo at the same time. I will have to do the chemo for one year. It is in a pill form called Temodor and is tolerated a lot easier than traditionally chemotherapy through an IV. It is more mild, has less side effects. Since it is pill form I will be able to be more flexible and get back to Portugal in July! :) My UCLA team is also working on putting together a Neuro team for me in Lisbon. When I am there I can do my scans and blood work which will be sent back to UCLA and we will all work together! Along with these treatments I will continue using all my holistic approaches especially the Keto diet, cannabis oil, frankincense oil, natural herbs and supplements. I will continue to use all these approaches for the rest of my life!! These tumors are brutal and never want to leave and stop growing. I will forever be on a mission to keep shrinking it and not let the monster continue to grow!

Let me also get straight to point and question I think many have, have asked, or don't want to ask…So does this mean you have cancer? Yes. Yes this means I have cancer, brain cancer, and have had it since the day I found out in January 2016. I also have most likely been living with this slow growing tumor in my brain for half my life. I guess I really didn't want to accept the fact I do indeed have brain cancer. I was hopeful and wanted to just be that amazing story of a girl that found out she had a brain tumor, had it removed and it never came back again.

Some other quick facts about brain tumors is that there is no cure so the tumor will never be 100% gone. So the fact there is no cure and they can never be resected 100% means I will most likely always have a brain tumor. The smaller that sucker the better and the main goal of all this is to keep the tumor small, stable and from growing. It wants to grow and it WILL grow, so the main objective is to do EVERYTHING possible to STOP it from growing back. I can live with a small brain tumor. In fact, today, an estimated 700,000 people in the United States are living with a primary brain tumor, and over 79,000 more will be diagnosed in 2018. Brain tumors can be deadly, significantly impact quality of life, and change everything for a patient and their loved ones. They do not discriminate, inflicting men, women and children of all races and ethnicities. The cause is completely unknown and that makes it impossible to prevent and extremely scary. Just stay aware of your own body and feelings and if something does not seem right then go to a doctor and get it checked out! Always better to be safe than sorry. I am also here for you and want to help with any questions I can. Especially if diagnosed, we are in this together and can get through it!!! I am positive, I am hopeful and I am going to kick this tumor's ass!!! Thank you for following my journey! I will keep you up to date on my treatments once they begin.

with love,

Kelsey

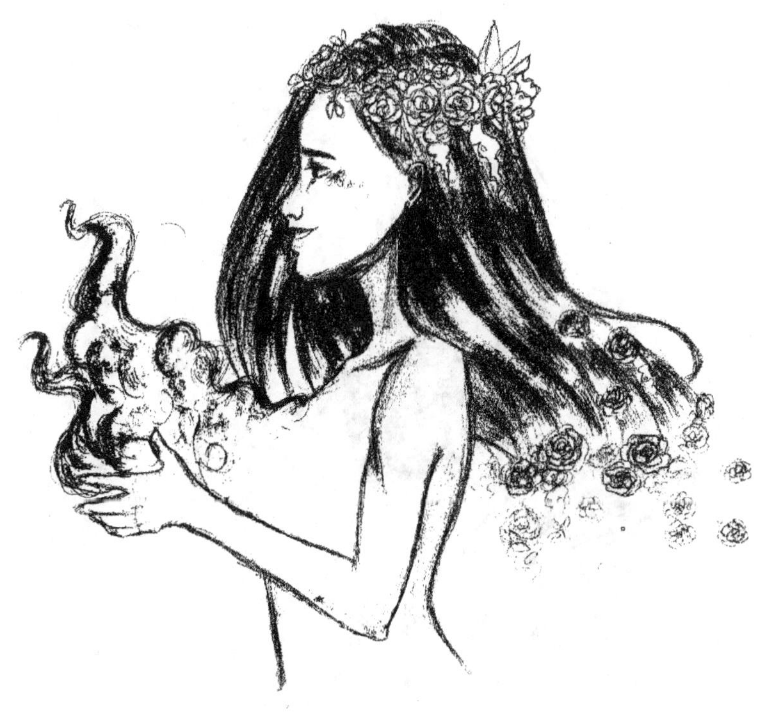

Sketch By Ellen Curtin

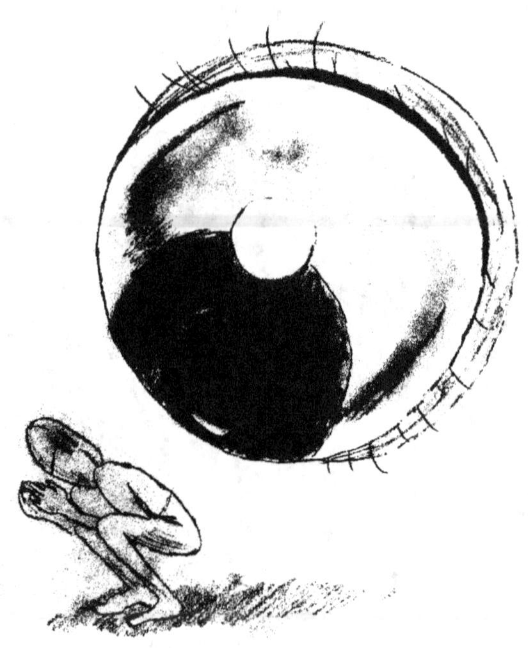

Sketch By Grace Wethor

<u>I</u>

all eyes are on you...
what are you gonna do......
what are you gonna change...........

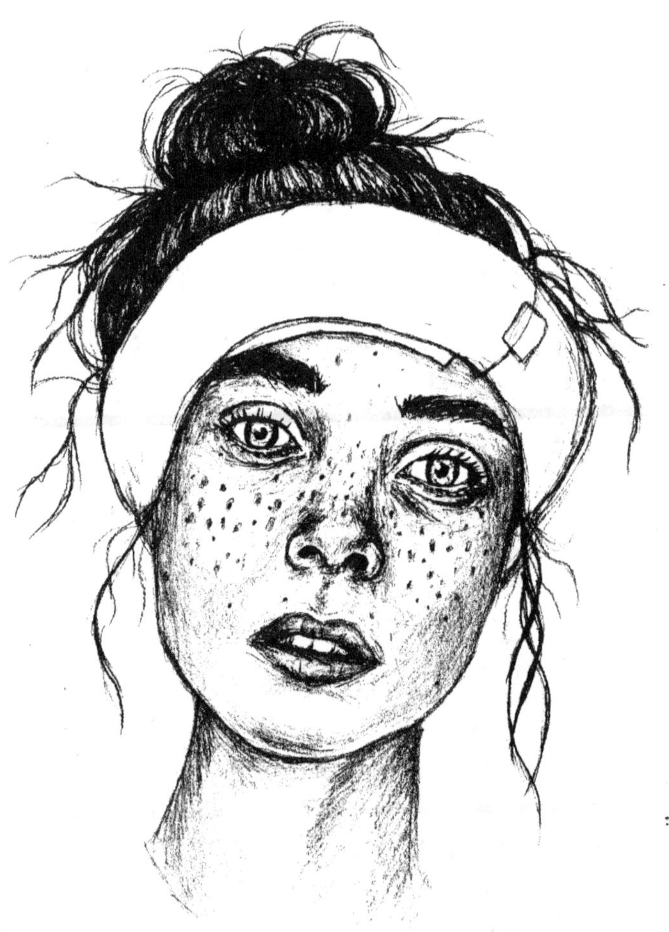

Sketch By Maryline Platevoet

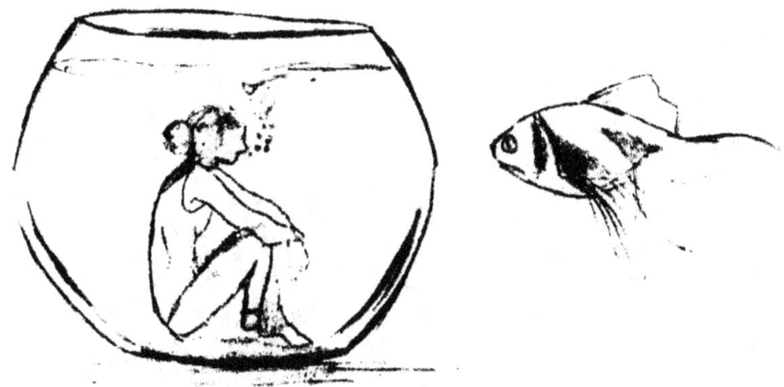

Sketch By Grace Wethor

Brooke Kotrla

Grade II Diffuse Astrocytoma Survivor

Brooke

People always ask me " how did you know you had a brain tumor?" or "what symptoms were you having?" I think it's mainly so they can self-diagnosis their headaches or other problems. I mean most people aren't thinking "I have a brain tumor" every time they have a headache. Well, maybe you do and if so you might be a hypochondriac so you should get some help for that! It all started a few years back when I was dancing. I've been dancing since I was a little girl. Let's start from there....

My parents were awesome and put me in all kinds of classes and activities as a kid. I did everything from cheerleading, gymnastics, dance and swimming. By the time I was about eight years old I started to realize I might have some talent for dance and I certainly had a passion for it. I spent all my time as a kid making up dance routines and I would force my family to watch them. My dad even built a stage in our basement for me! In middle school I would sit at home after school (before dance classes) and watch Youtube videos of college dance teams. I watched videos of other dancers in order to learn and make myself better. I stalked competitive college dance teams online to see who was the best and I was determined to be on one of those teams one day. By the time I was in high school, I had danced at a summer intensive with the Joffrey Ballet Jazz group in Miami and taken some classes in L.A. and of course with companies in downtown Chicago, which is where I lived at the time. My dance teachers had been encouraging me for a while to attend a performing arts high school and even talked to my mom about how I would flourish in that kind of environment.

I started high school in Chicago and was continuing to take excessive amounts of dance classes weekly. I was also on the Varsity POM/Dance team at my high school. I took jazz, hiphop, modern, contemporary, ballet, acro-dance, and pointe. I was also competing in dance competitions with my dance company after school regionally and nationally. In 2012 my MiMi, who I was very close with, passed away from cancer at a young age of 63. She fought Leukemia hard but lost her battle quickly as her disease progressed rapidly once she was diagnosed. This made a strong impact on me and made me want to pursue my dreams even more and dance for her.

Later that year, after talking to my parents, I applied to Houston's High School for the Performing and Visual Arts (HSPVA) dance program and was accepted. It was a dream come true yet we would have to move. I didn't mind that much because I love change and to me moving is more exciting than scary. I'd miss all my Chicago dance friends, but I was also so excited to get the chance to move to Houston. My brother was a senior in high school in Chicago and I would be a sophomore in Houston. We all sacrificed to fulfill my dream. My mom quit her job and we moved together to Houston that year. My dad and brother now had the "bachelor pad" we called it, which was our house in Chicago. My brother, Blake, lived out his senior year and searched for colleges. My dad put our house on the market to sell once he graduated. It was a stressful year but also full of wonderful memories. My mom and I loved spending time together and we made great memories that year. It was a radical change from living in the suburbs of Chicago but my grandparents lived in Houston so it was very familiar and felt like home in many ways.

By the end of my sophomore year I had grown so much as a dancer at HSPVA. My brother graduated high school and my dad moved to Houston to be with us. My parents made such a sacrifice for my dance career. They both left jobs to come to Houston with no employment to allow me to dance at HSPVA in order to fulfill a life-long dream. It's kind of crazy when you think about it! But it wasn't a blind sacrifice. We felt that God was leading us to move to Houston for this opportunity even though is didn't quite make sense. I've found that God often calls us to things before he provides the way.

My parents both got great jobs and we bought a house in the suburbs. My brother somewhat reluctantly decided to go to college in Texas in order to not be so far away from the family and I danced after school at one of the best and most competitive companies in Texas. I danced every day in school, after school, weekends with my company, and numerous competitions. I was blessed to be on a team that won national dance competitions in jazz and lyrical dance which are my two strongest styles.

My senior year was filled with college visits, dance clinics, and auditioning for dance programs. I was finally almost able to touch my dream. The time had come. I even worked with a private coach during the fall semester to help me hone some of my skills I knew some of the teams would be looking for. This way I was in the best shape possible and ready for tryouts.

After looking at numerous schools, Texas Tech's program was my number one choice… if I could get a spot on the highly competitive team. Many girls were returning to the team so I wasn't sure if there would be many spots open. Auditions were in April. I went through the first interview round and one of the Public Relations people asked me what conference Texas Tech was in and I said, "the SEC?" hesitantly. Of course, I was wrong. It's the Big 12…I felt like an idiot because I knew nothing about football. I hope I hadn't already blown it!

The next day were dance auditions and cuts came every few hours. I made it to the final round the third day but a small group of girls were pulled back for a separate look. That is never a good thing in auditions…. I was so nervous. That was the last item on the audition itinerary after three days and then we waited anxiously about two hours for a text message to be posted. That afternoon my dream was realized! I had made the dream team I had been working for since I was little girl. I was on a Big 12 conference dance team and would represent the university at all sporting events on television, fundraisers, social media, and with the National Dance Alliance college competitive dance teams.

My freshman year at Texas Tech in many ways was a dream come true and filled with many once in a lifetime experiences. Mixed in with all of this were the start of what we now know may have been signs of my growing brain tumor. Thanksgiving that year (2015) I was living in the dorm and was running high fever, had terrible headaches, and trouble moving my neck. My mom thought I had meningitis at first.   After seeing doctors at the school health clinic, urgent care, the ER, and finally at home over break we found out I had mono. It took months for me to recover from the energy loss. I really didn't feel like myself until later that spring. I remember crying at home because I didn't want to go back for the spring semester. School and my dance team were becoming mentally and emotionally draining.

By the end of that semester I still felt like I needed a break. The demands for the POM dance team are very heavy and I felt like I couldn't keep up if I tried out again. Learning multiple routines all the time requires a great amount of focus and looking back I think my brain struggled through this. I remember specifically how I enjoyed just going to the gym and working out because it didn't require me to focus on anything and it wasn't hard.

Not trying out for the POM team again was one of the hardest decisions I have ever made. My coaches didn't understand. They were losing a strong dancer and team member. Some of my friends felt betrayed. Even my parents didn't understand how their daughter who had been striving for this goal for 10 years and achieved it would walk away after one year. My mom couldn't wrap her head around my decision but was supportive when I told her I didn't want to do another year. Once that decision was made I decided to go to Texas State University to be with my brother. Blake was a senior and I could be closer to home. I would focus on my fitness career now which I really enjoyed.

Little did I know things were changing. That summer after POM I set out to do a bikini fitness competition and placed first in my category! I had worked so hard and it felt good. But after that, I knew some things were not right in my body. I hadn't had my period most of the year prior while on Texas Tech POM and not recently either while prepping for my fitness competition.

My mom took me to the gynecologist who diagnosed with me with polycystic ovaries (PCOS) and said I probably should be on birth control pills. I started on them in August and within 60 days I had gained almost 20 pounds. Which for a 5'2" girl (or anyone) is A LOT of weight. By Thanksgiving (90 days) I had gained more weight and was having increasing headaches. After discussing with my mom, we agreed I should get off the pills. Christmas 2016 rolled around and I was still having some headaches. They went on throughout the spring as well. Even with a more strict diet and still continuing to work out regularly, I had trouble losing the weight I had gained

Spring 2017 was the defining point that led to my diagnosis. Over those months while at school, I was increasingly lethargic. I would get up, eat breakfast, go to class, workout, and come back to my apartment and sleep. I rarely ever went out or met up with friends. I was alive but I wasn't even living because I just felt so weird. I started having visual problems and would see rainbows in my peripheral vision. My right arm would occasionally tingle. I would feel like my body was floating in outer space. It was especially scary when I was driving. These were all random symptoms so none of it really made sense. I thought the vision problems might be associated with my headaches like an aura and migraines. By the end of the semester my headaches had increased and I was having trouble moving my neck side to side. My whole body was just off. Considering in the past six months all my weight gain, headaches, vision and tingling problems. It was hard for me to even understand what was happening with my body.

I came home after spring finals and my parents sent me to the chiropractor and to get my eyes checked. The eye doctor said the optic nerves in both my eyes were swollen and that I needed to see a neurologist to make sure everything was ok. My mom, being a nurse, knew that was not normal so she called the eye doctor that day and asked if this was an emergency since we couldn't get an appointment for two weeks. She said no but it needs to be soon.

That was the day before the Memorial Day weekend 2017. Throughout the weekend I iced my neck, took ibuprofen and Tylenol, and slept most of the weekend. I passed up opportunities to go to master dance classes with my friends who were also home from college and I missed pool parties for the holiday. My mom was worried about the way I was acting. Even my two best friends came over to see me and commented that I looked sick.

The day after the Memorial Day holiday, my parents took me to the ER. I was taking a nap and my mom came to wake me up and said she thinks we shouldn't wait to see the neurologist and should get checked out sooner. She knew there could be more going on. She tells people now that she was watching me suffer and go down hill day after day that weekend and couldn't sit still any longer.

At the ER, we told them about what the eye doctor said and that I probably needed an MRI and to see a neurologist. I had my first of many MRIs that day, May 30, 2017. My life was forever changed an hour later.

The ER doctor came in and told us there was a mass and they needed to send us via ambulance to a neurosurgeon down in the Houston Medical Center. They said they were not sure if I needed surgery tonight or not but it was urgent. They started giving me IV steroids immediately for the swelling in my head. My parents and I were in a state of shock. In the whirlwind of shock, fear, and disbelief my mom told the ER doctor that she didn't want to go to their hospital. She needed to make some calls first. We have a friend who lost her husband to a brain tumor years back and they started a foundation that supports brain cancer research at MD Anderson Cancer Center. The Broach Foundation for Brain Cancer Research is one of the largest donors to brain cancer research at MD Anderson. My mom called her in the middle of the night and she reached out to their head neuro-surgeon and lead researcher, Dr Fred Lang. Dr. Lang called my mom within five minutes and asked her to text a picture of my MRI. He said he would meet us at MD Anderson ER as soon as the ambulance could get there. Unfortunately, I was not a patient there so the ER is not open to me and the ambulance would not take me there. Dr. Lang got on the phone with the ER doctor and after about 45 minutes of paperwork and discussion I was on my way.

It was my first and hopefully last ambulance ride at 2am in the morning. Dr. Lang and my mom's friend met us there in the ER that night. He immediately took us to a room and started to talk to us about what was next. I also vividly remember a nurse gave me a sandwich- so I knew this would be a good hospital once the food started coming. Who doesn't like a sandwich at 2am? I was admitted to the hospital for a few days to monitor me and for excessive amounts of tests on my brain. I had MRIs of every kind to make a GPS map of my brain and my tumor. I did hand motions and spoke the names of images on cards while machines mapped out my brain activity. My brain felt fried at the end of all the tests. It left me so tired and worn down after all the MRI tests. I was put on pain medications and a seizure medication as a precaution and sent home a few days later. My surgery was planned for four days later.

Going home was the worst time ever. I had all the time in the world to think about my massive brain surgery that was ahead of me. Dr. Lang wanted a special anesthesiologist that could manage me being awake for the surgery as much as possible. Thinking about my skull being open and someone taking out my brain tumor freaked me out. I was so stressed and scared the few days before my surgery. The only thing I had to do was watch Netflix. Dr. Lang and Dr. Ferson were the best in the field and I needed to remember that. Dr. Ferson, the anesthesiologist, who I remember seeing throughout my surgery and he held my hand. We met them ahead of time and they made me feel more comfortable.

My surgery was June 8, 2017. I had an awake craniotomy that lasted over 10 hours. I was awake for four of those hours. After the surgery, we found out I had 34 seizures during the operation. It was possibly historic in nature due to the number of them and made the surgery somewhat difficult at times for Dr. Lang. I remember hearing him during the procedure saying "Are you kidding…she's having another one?!?" The best way to stop a seizure during a craniotomy is to pour cold water straight on to your brain. People ask me all the time if I remember the surgery and I emphatically say, "Yes!" I remember the sounds, the images, the voices, and some of the seizures. I remember the pouring of cold water on my brain and the pain that caused me. The cold water calms the seizing nerves but also freezes other nerves like the ones in the back of your throat. I remember my face shaking and my neck seizing. I was fully aware I was having a seizure but my body laid their unable to respond. What I don't remember is what came after. I don't remember almost five days in the ICU, all the pain my parents say I experienced and had to be medicated for, all the medication side effects, and all the things I was hooked up to for days to monitor my brain activity, blood pressure, brain drainage, EKG, IVs, etc. I do remember people who visited, however. I also remember the scriptures we had posted on my hospital room walls to remind us of God's faithfulness and power that is bigger than cancer.

It was one of the most difficult times for all of us. I was diagnosed with a grade 2 diffuse astrocytoma immediately post op but we had to wait on final pathology a few weeks to know more. The surgeons were not optimistic because my tumor did not test positive for a certain mutation that is common in these low grade tumors called IDH1. It generally is seen first thing on the pathology report but it did not show up on mine. The doctors said if you don't have it your tumor is called a "wild type" and can be more difficult to treat as they can't determine how treatment regimes respond and the outcomes are much less favorable. My mom knew all of this but I was still so focused on my recovery for the weeks following my surgery. I didn't know or pay attention to what all of that meant. I am glad I didn't know this at the time or I would have been even more stressed out… I was still needing pain medication for a few weeks after, was on steroids for swelling for weeks, and now was on three different seizure meds.

Weeks later in July, I was preparing to start six weeks of proton radiation and my mom came into the room crying. My full genetics testing had come back and they found the IDH1 mutation. It was hiding there all along! It was a more rare type of it that could only be found through a full DNA panel and the genetics people had to go hunting for it. My oncologist said this was a "very good day!" We all cried that day knowing that God is always at work despite what the situation looks like on the surface.

July 12, 2017 I started my six weeks of daily proton therapy. I am so blessed to have been approved for proton radiation. It is a superior type of radiation because it focuses high beams of energy into your tumor. The energy is shot into your tumor from one side and mysteriously is doesn't come out the other side like X-rays do or traditional radiation. The catch is that you have to wear a custom made mouth guard and mask over your whole head that is then strapped down to the proton table. It is so precise they even take an X-ray every day once you are strapped down to make sure it is within 1mm accurate. I guess you don't want them zapping the wrong parts, right! The treatments lasted 25-30 minutes so you can't move and barely breathe. It is pretty annoying but I did have a great radiation team and they would play whatever music you wanted in the room to make the time go by as quick as possible. My parents would also sit in the waiting room and would send snapchats so when I got out there were crazy pics on my phone. I always had radiation late at night so all those snapchats were of my delirious friends and family who would wait for me to be done.

One thing no one knows about proton radiation of the brain is that you see or smell things that aren't there when the radiation is being shot into your head. The doctors told me this would happen so I expected it but it is still weird when you think about it. They said it is because the brain is receiving a signal that is does not know what to do with so it takes the closest thing and makes up an interpretation. I had four directions (or fields) to get my radiation so whenever the proton ray would change directions I would know because I knew which one gave me the sense of seeing blue and purple lights or I would smell plastic or eggs. I mean why couldn't I smell roses or chocolate chip cookies? I always knew which field they were doing because of the vision or smells.

At the end of 30 rounds of radiation they give you a ceremony and you ring a huge gong after your last treatment. My friends and family were there and they played "Miracles Happen" from the Princess Diaries when I walked out of the room. That song always makes me feel happy. Honestly, anything Disney makes me happy. I signed a giant wall of other survivors, we took pictures with beautiful flowers, and then went for dessert after. The best medication around!

My doctors told me they would allow a rest of 2-3 weeks before I had to start my year long chemo. In the meantime, I had a few things to do. First they wanted me to see a fertility oncologist to consider preserving my eggs. I guess I had never thought of this but I am glad they did. We met with Dr. Woodard and her staff. They were so nice and walked us through the whole process. To be honest I did not like it and dreaded the whole thing but I knew it was something in needed to do for my future. It is also a very expensive process and not covered by insurance so I was happy to have some help from the LIVESTRONG Fertility Foundation.

Second, during that three week break I had always wanted a tattoo and felt this was the perfect time to get one. I had just turned 21 during my last few weeks of proton therapy and knew I couldn't get one while on chemo for the next year. I decided I wanted a rose and I wanted to get it together with my mom. I have never been a big flower person but ever since I had my surgery I have loved flowers so much more. I looked to the Bible for inspiration for my tattoo. A rose symbolizes the beauty in life or death, because we are saved by the One

True King. I read this quote, "How precious are my children who are awed by natures beauty; this opens them up to my Holy Presence." The more I reach toward God the more I notice the beauty of His presence in the small things in the world.

Hurricane Harvey happened during my three week treatment break so that put a damper on things significantly. We evacuated our house for a few days and it delayed my egg retrieval start a bit. Once we survived the flood, my flood of hormones began. I had to get multiple shots in my abdomen at night daily to grow my eggs and then get blood drawn and an ultrasound every 48 hours to watch the eggs grow. It is IVF for the purposes of getting out as many eggs as possible to freeze for later. Because I am only 21, I was very responsive to the hormones they gave me and my ovaries were almost hyper-stimulated. They had to watch them very closely. Long story short, after two weeks of this painful process and feeling like I was pregnant …I couldn't even light my favorite candle because it made me nauseous….they removed 29 eggs! A typical, successful egg retrieval gets about 10-15 eggs. 29!!! That is over two years of periods AT ONE TIME. My fertility doctor said I have over-achieving ovaries and my mom told her I never did anything half-way LOL!

I was so glad that was over and considered that having brain surgery might have been easier than having to go through that again…probably not… but I did consider the idea. The week after that I was invited to Texas Tech to be on the field for a football game with my team. I hoped I had the energy to make it through the whole day as I was still recovering from radiation fatigue and the IVF had really knocked me out. They showered me with love, gifts and hugs! It was a sweet reunion to see everyone but I was still pretty tired. My mom brought me Starbucks with an espresso shot halfway through the day to give me a boost of energy thankfully and I had to sit down on the sidelines through the game but the energy and adrenaline kept me going.

I returned home to start my first round of 12 months of chemo. I wasn't sure what to expect. My chemotherapy is a pill so thankfully I take it at home at night before I go to bed for one week. I am now six months into my chemotherapy regime and know much better what to expect and how to address it. My go-tos for nausea are Seabands, Zofran, peppermint oil, and puppy snuggles. I basically have to sleep a lot during my treatments to keep me from feeling the worst and it makes me super tired. Also walking around makes me feel sicker as well so being still helps.

I get brain MRIs every 60 days now. Immediately after radiation I was getting them every 30 days to watch an enhanced spot that came up on the first MRI. The doctors call it a pseudo-progression and say it is common right after radiation because it has messed with your tumor cells so much. That spot has changed slightly over the past few MRIs but nothing drastic so we continue to watch and wait. All in all, my team is pleased with my progress thus far. As am I! Sometimes I wonder if I will ever be cancer free. I've gotten to the place where I don't care about that as much. As long as it is controlled and I can live my life I'm fine with it.

I am currently a junior in college and between my chemo treatments I do school through Texas Tech online and try to eat well and exercise. I am really getting into Pilates reformer classes lately. Have you tried this? It is super challenging and not for the faint of heart! I want to stay as active as possible. Fitness has always been important to me even before my diagnosis. Right after my surgery there were things I could not do or were too weak for. Since then I haven't had any restrictions or problems with doing any type of activity I want to do thankfully. I've started dancing again too and love how moving makes me feel. As I think about my future I can't say exactly what I want to do but I know I want to make a positive impact on people's lives. I might end up doing something in fitness, dance, or in a health-related field.

What I know about cancer is that it changes your life forever but it is not all for the worst. I am learning what really matters most. My relationship with God has grown tremendously. I've learned who my real friends are and who truly loves me through sickness and health and through baldness and full hair! I am learning to be more present in my life. I cry more than ever but I don't care anymore because it means that I am alive and I feel deeply. I've learned I have a strong sense of injustice and want what is right for everyone especially those fighting cancer. I have recognized I am a positive, determined, and more courageous person than I knew and I want to use those strengths for good. And finally I've learned that cancer is only a part of my life but not all of who I am. I would never wish cancer on anyone. Not even my worst enemy. I do wish others could see what it teaches you as a person. As humans we get so wrapped up in life that we forget to really live and love in it. You can always make a change if you're not happy. Cancer sucks but I'm so lucky to have turned this into a positive learning experience. The worst thing you can do is sit around and be a negative nancy soaking in all the negative parts of your life. I could do that too but I know that was not how we were intended to live our lives.

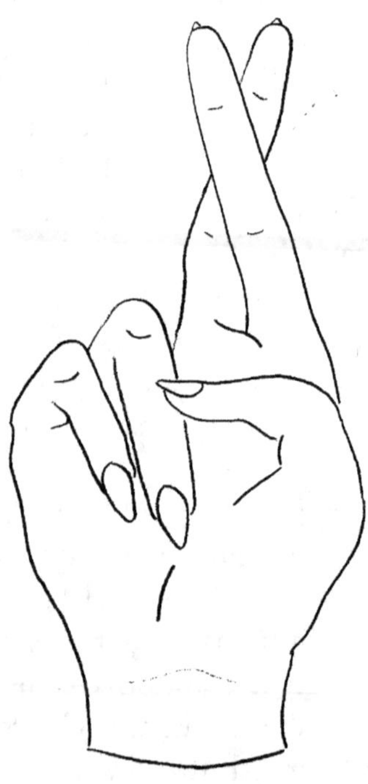

CLOSING REMARKS

I don't know what's next for me...
I don't know what my future holds...
from a treatment standpoint and from a life standpoint.

Right now I continue to monitor my tumor with MRIs and hope that the future holds some form of treatment for my type of tumor. I still deal with symptoms on a daily basis, but am learning to handle them and look at them with a positive mindset. I focus on living my life to the fullest and not taking any day for granted. I truly believe that doing the things I love is the reason I passed my expected survival date.

I don't know if I consider myself "lucky", I still haven't decided...and I think that's okay. One thing I know for sure is that life can change in an instant, and deciding to do the things you love and live the life you want...well... it might just save you...

Grace Ash Wethor

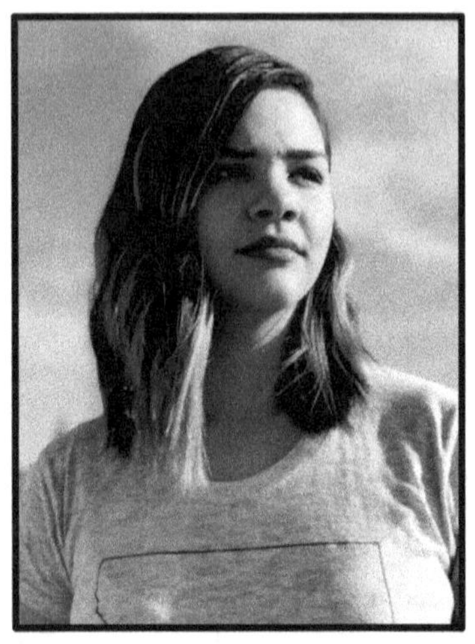

Gabrielle Camacho
Survivor, 16
Los Angeles, CA

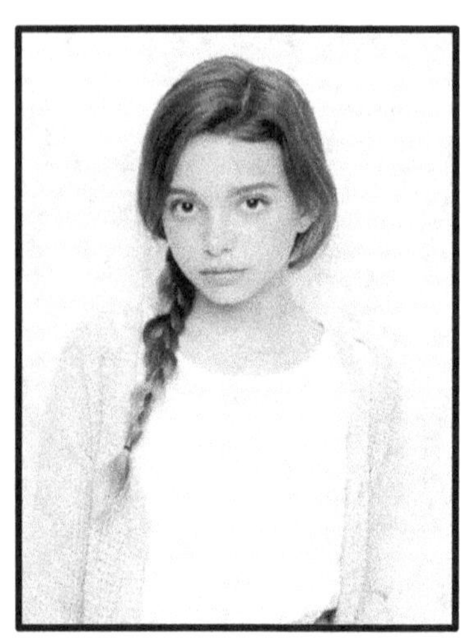

Alexa Ponciano
Survivor, 15
San Fransisco, CA

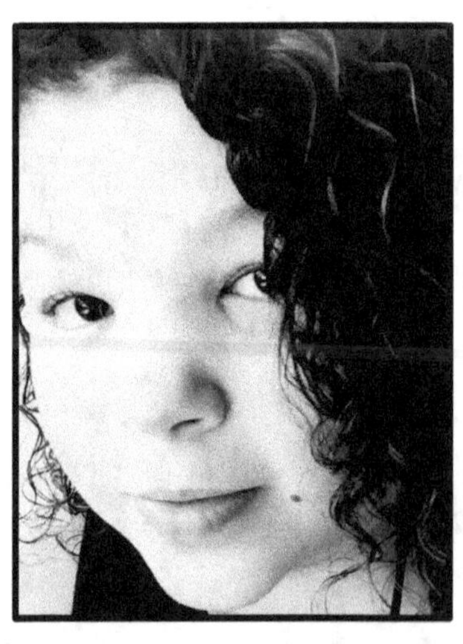

Sierra Barnes
Survivor, 21
Dallas, TX

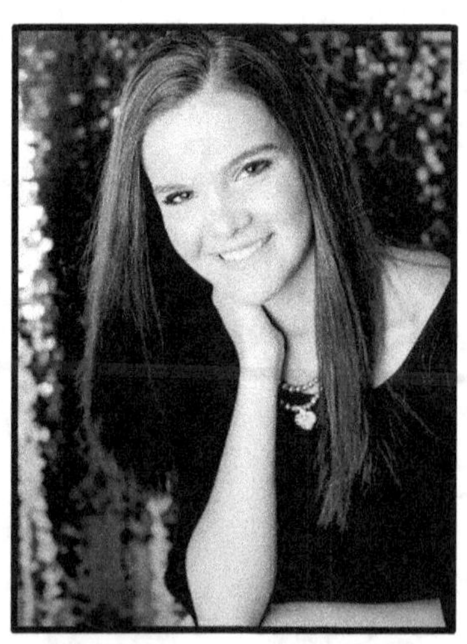

Madison Williams
Survivor, 18
Flowery Branch, GA

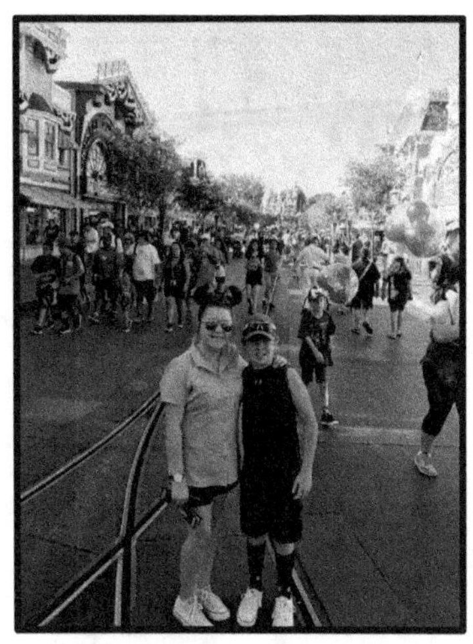

Miki A.R.
Survivor, 15
Huffman, TX

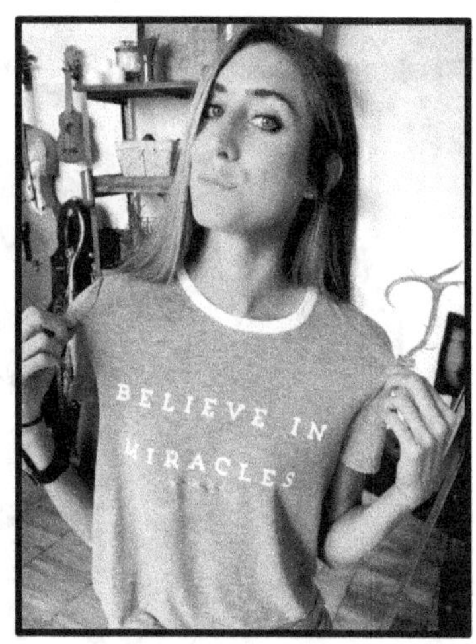

Erin Elizabeth
Survivor, 28
Chicago, IL

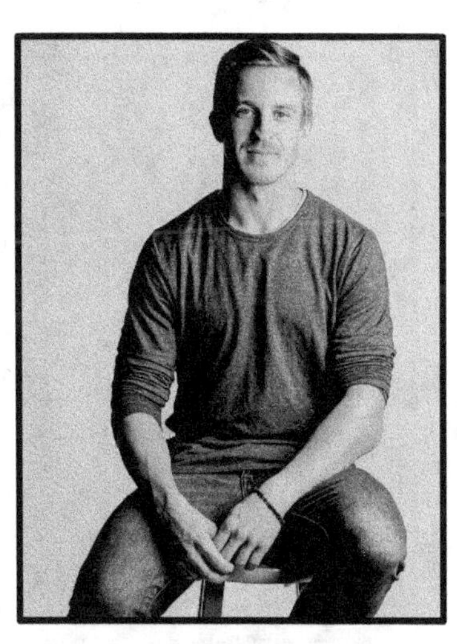

Josh Perry
Survivor, 29
Raleigh, NC

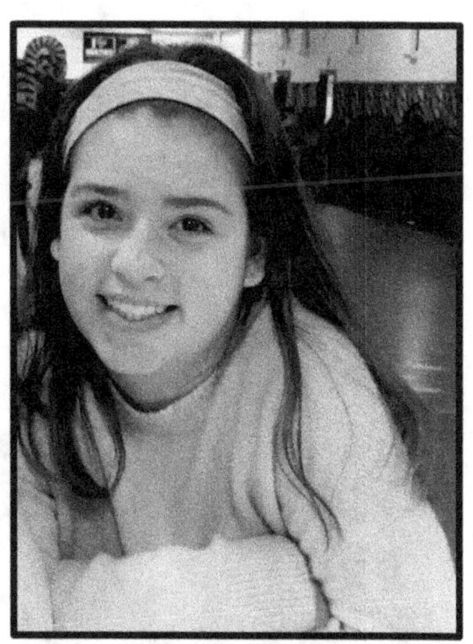

Meghan Pawlak
Survivor, 14
Buffalo, NY

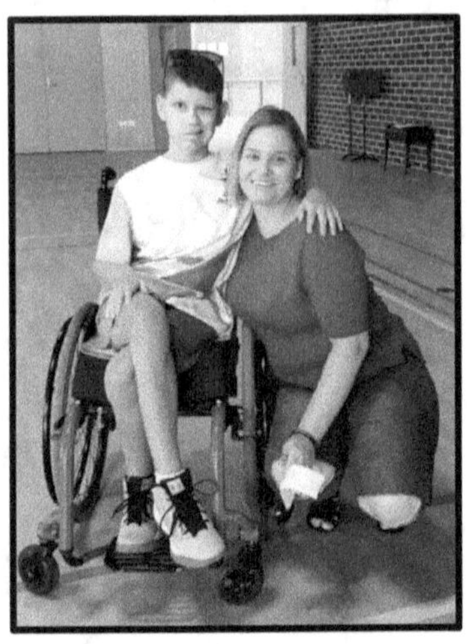

Suzanne Turpie
Mother of Survivor
Port Macquarie, Australia

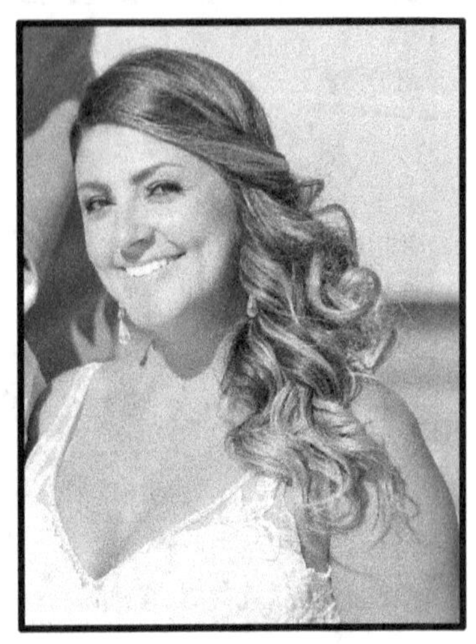

Kelsey Taveira
Survivor, 32
Portimão, Portugal &
Redondo Beach, CA

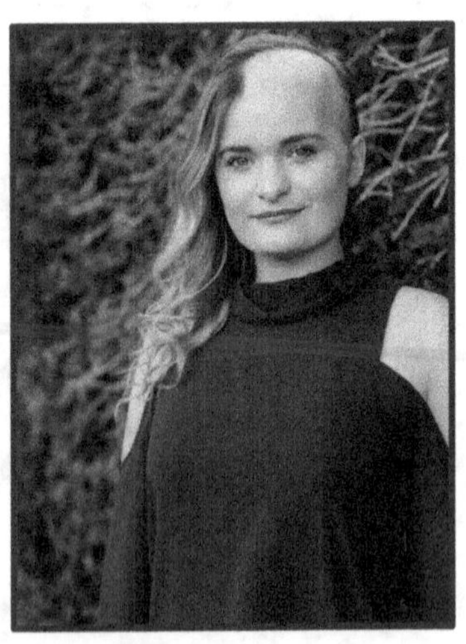

Brooke Kotrla
Survivor, 21
Huston, TX

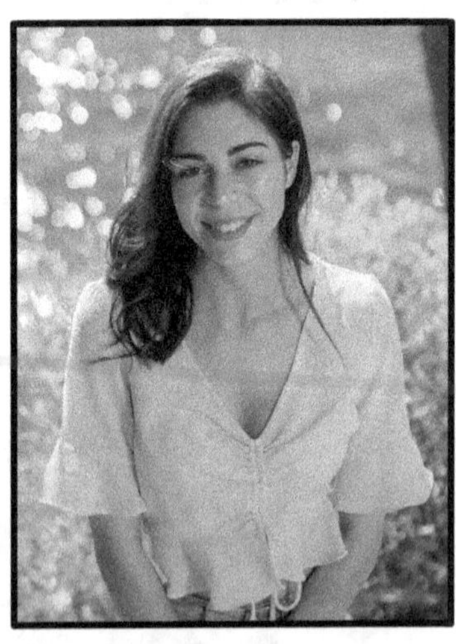

Heather Rosati
Illustrator, 17
San Diego, CA

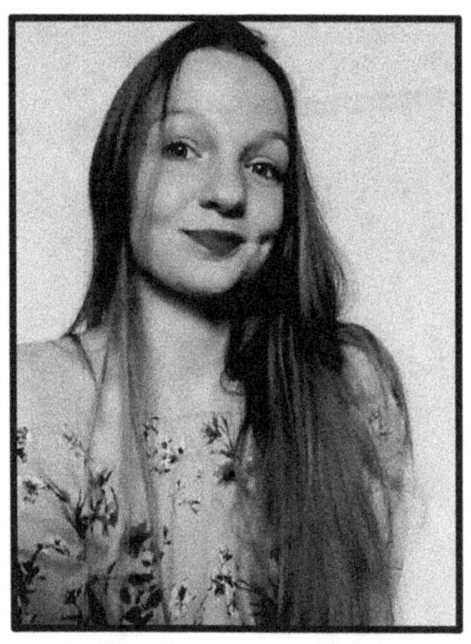

Maryline Platevoet
Illustrator, 19
Lille, France

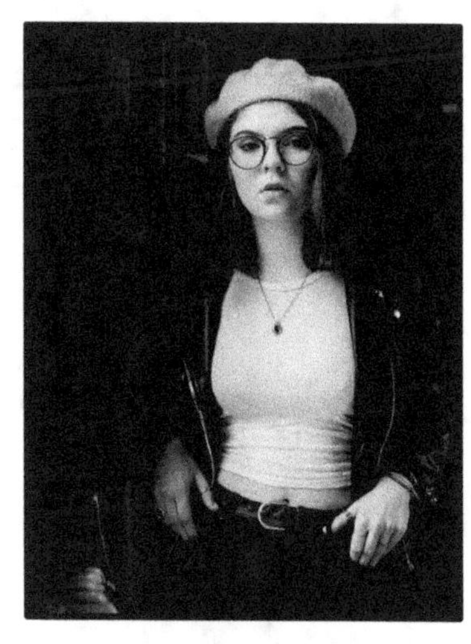

Jaiden Bjorklund
Illustrator, 17
Minneapolis, MN

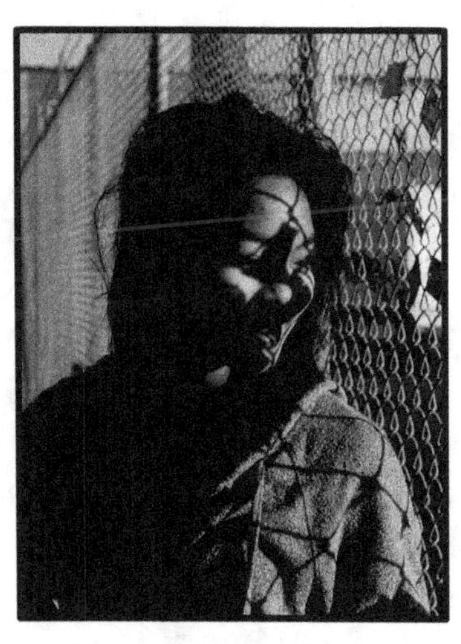

Ellen Curtin
Illustrator, 17
Minneapolis, MN

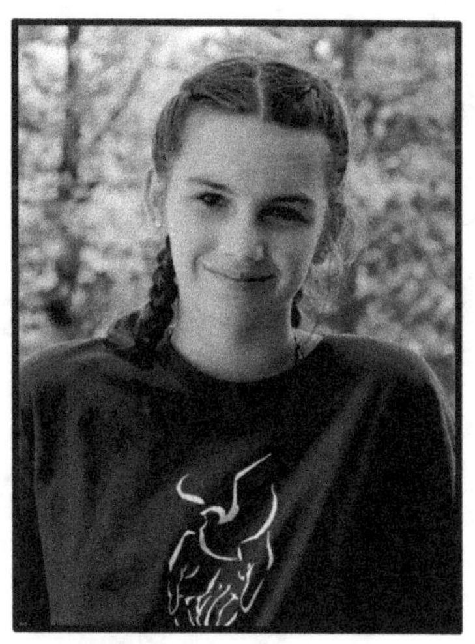

Rachel Kramer
Illustrator, 15
Carlsbad, CA

Content Edited By
Alex Lodner

The information in this book is not intended or implied to be a substitute for professional medical advice, diagnosis or treatment. All content, including text, graphics, images, discussions and information, contained in this book is for general information purposes only. The authors, contributors and hosts make no representation and assume no responsibility for the accuracy of information contained, and such information is subject to change without notice. You are encouraged to confirm any information obtained from or through this book and/or related discussions with other sources and review all information regarding any medical condition or treatment with your physician. NEVER DISREGARD PROFESSIONAL MEDICAL ADVICE OR DELAY SEEKING MEDICAL TREATMENT BECAUSE OF SOMETHING YOU HAVE READ IN OR ACCESSED THROUGH THIS BOOK OR RELATED DISCUSSIONS.